The Public Health Nurses of Jim Crow Florida

D1522055

UNIVERSITY PRESS OF FLORIDA

Florida A&M University, Tallahassee
Florida Atlantic University, Boca Raton
Florida Gulf Coast University, Ft. Myers
Florida International University, Miami
Florida State University, Tallahassee
New College of Florida, Sarasota
University of Central Florida, Orlando
University of Florida, Gainesville
University of North Florida, Jacksonville
University of South Florida, Tampa
University of West Florida, Pensacola

THE PUBLIC HEALTH NURSES OF
||||||||||||||||||||||||||||||||||||||||||||||||||||||||||||||||||||||||||||||||||||||||||
JIM CROW FLORIDA
||||||||||||||||||||||||||||||||||||||||||||||||||||||||||||||||||||||||||||||||||||||||||

Christine Ardalan

UNIVERSITY PRESS OF FLORIDA

Gainesville / Tallahassee / Tampa / Boca Raton

Pensacola / Orlando / Miami / Jacksonville / Ft. Myers / Sarasota

Library of Congress Cataloging-in-Publication Data
Names: Ardalan, Christine, author.
Title: The public health nurses of Jim Crow Florida / Christine Ardalan.
Description: Gainesville, FL : University Press of Florida, [2019] | Includes
    bibliographical references and index.
Identifiers: LCCN 2019004285 | ISBN 9780813066158 (cloth : alk. paper) | ISBN
    9780813068589 (pbk.)
Subjects: LCSH: Nursing—Florida—History—20th century. | Health services
    accessibility—Florida.
Classification: LCC RT5.F6 A73 2019 | DDC 610.7309759—dc23
LC record available at https://lccn.loc.gov/2019004285

The University Press of Florida is the scholarly publishing agency for the State
University System of Florida, comprising Florida A&M University, Florida Atlantic
University, Florida Gulf Coast University, Florida International University, Florida
State University, New College of Florida, University of Central Florida, University
of Florida, University of North Florida, University of South Florida, and University
of West Florida.

University Press of Florida
2046 NE Waldo Road
Suite 2100
Gainesville, FL 32609
http://upress.ufl.edu

Contents

Figures

Acknowledgments

The seeds of this book sprouted unknowingly during my nurse training at King's College Hospital in London—but grew much later when I immigrated and became hooked on English and history classes at the University of Miami and Florida International University. The cultural context of nurses' work captured my interest and nourished my path in Florida. Along the way, many nurses and others in the medical, academic, and lay communities have encouraged me, supported me, and helped me understand the complexities of nursing and midwifery practice during the Jim Crow era in Florida. I am deeply grateful to them all.

I extend my heartfelt thanks to Thelma Gibson for sharing her experiences with me more than twenty years ago; she opened a path for me to reach into the African American community by introducing me to colleagues who also willingly shared their stories. My oral history research was enhanced by support from the Florida Humanities Council; Dorothy Fields, the founder of Miami's Black Archives; and Mary Elizabeth Carnegie, a powerhouse who fought for racial justice in nursing and mentored Florida's African American nurses. Thus, my work took on a community dimension, and I feel especially indebted not only to the interviewees and new friends like Gail VanderVoort but also to the late Arva Moore Parks and the late William M. Straight. I am profoundly thankful that Arva and Bill offered their insights into local and state history, and Bill passed along a wealth of information about medical history as well. Now, thanks to collaboration with Vicki Silvera, the head of Special Collections at Florida International University, Bill's medical collection has a home.

This book's focus on the historical context of public health nursing in Florida benefited from Kirsten Wood's outstanding support and insight. Darden

Pyron, Sherry Johnson, David Cook, and Joyce Peterson also deepened my scholarship and deserve my sincere gratitude. Helping me to expand my research more broadly, Patsy West shared her research and knowledge about Native American culture. Kim Curry, Katherine Mason, Charlton Praether, and the late Dolores Wennlund sharpened my focus on public health. And digging into the nursing history of the American Red Cross has been one of the joys of my archival research, particularly when aided by the nurse researcher for the American Red Cross Jean Waldman Shulman. Her willingness to impart her broad nursing scholarship extended to her companionship on our many research missions that were such a great pleasure.

My thanks also go to Giselle Roberts and Melissa Walker, who accepted my contribution of the first state health nurses' work for their book centered on southern women in the Progressive Era and encouraged me to complete my study. For the refocus and reworking of the manuscript, I owe Sian Hunter, the senior editor of the University Press of Florida, my wholehearted gratitude for her input and the meaningful ways she helped me to improve it. The final book would not have come to fruition without her suggestions and help. I am also grateful to Dr. James Crook as well as the anonymous reviewers for their comments and suggestions that I believe have also strengthened the manuscript.

Finally, from the deepest place in my heart I want to thank my husband, Bach; our children, Katherine, Mark, Georgina, and Joanna; my daughter-in-law, Christine; and my sister, Ruth, for their love, support, and patience throughout the time I have been working toward this book. I greatly appreciate that they have all so willingly accompanied my journey.

Introduction

Opening a New Profession for
Women in Florida, 1914 to 1964

Set during the Jim Crow era, this book centers on Florida's public health nurses, mostly white and a few black women, who tackled the state's public health issues born of race, climate, geography, and poverty. These pioneering professional women were often the only ones available to take the messages of health improvement into the homes of people who were out of the reach of modern medical care. From the Panhandle to the Everglades and on to the Florida Keys, these nurses faced a number of challenges beginning with reaching both white and African American citizens in rural communities. Once the nurses arrived in remote homesteads, they had to translate scientific facts and medical perspectives into the idiom and context of these particular people who were shaped by nonmedical and nonscientific beliefs and behaviors. "Country people are . . . accustomed to slow thinking. . . . They are not so accustomed to interference with their plans or suggestions regarding changes that might be beneficial," wrote Laurie Jean Reid (1884–1958), the director of the Bureau of Child Welfare and public health nursing for the State Board of Health of Florida from 1922 to 1929.[1] Public health nurses had to find innovative ways to bridge the communities they served with the state and national public health policies that addressed the threats of infection and the high infant and maternal mortality levels. As Surgeon General Thomas Parran pointed out in 1938, they were the vital link in the "three-horse team of doctor, nurse and citizen" and bore "the brunt of the battle" to bring public health measures into the communities.[2]

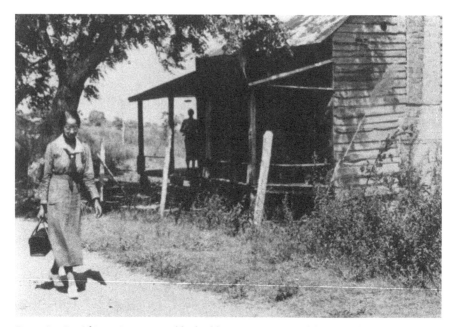

Figure I.1. An African American public health nurse visits a rural home in the South, ca. 1920. Courtesy of the National Library of Medicine.

Competing cultural constructions of health shaped their ground-breaking efforts to reach and serve underprivileged folk of all races, whether to prevent illness and disease or improve childbirth and general well-being.

As pioneering professional women in a state where white supremacy formed the bedrock of society, the women's roles as public health nurses gave them status and purpose to connect with communities, work around the cultural mores, and complete their missions. They drew strength from their professional identity, but it was also their personalities and the sheer force of their characters that served them in meeting the particular cultural and environmental challenges that set Florida apart from its northern neighbors. Strong characters were vital if the nurses were to travel the state alone and negotiate the environmental and cultural obstacles. The conditions prompted Reid to implore Florida's own professional white nurses to take up the mantle of public health nursing. She declared that only those familiar with the state would understand the demands. "It is difficult for nurses from the North to know individual problems of Florida," she told a local newspaper in 1922.[3]

Many black professional northern nurses were very aware of the "individual problem" of working in Florida or any other southern state. According to one black national nurse leader, Rosa Williams Brown (b. 1888), who arrived in Jacksonville from New York in 1914, motivated professional black nurses were well suited to meet Florida's needs. "We could see the needs of . . . our people as no one else could," she stated.[4] While Reid initially cracked open the door for one black nurse to join the staff, in a blatant show of racism the State Board of Health would not continue her employment. It took black nurses a double dose of resolve to face Florida's cultural roadblocks in their professional lives. For Brown, it took fifteen years before she could take up local public health work in the neglected African American community of West Palm Beach. To be sure, while both black and white nurses were active agents for change, cultural mores informed their practices differently. Professional patterns and social customs influenced the routes and manner they could exert power and influence to literally save people's lives.

The work of Florida's public health nurses underscores the importance of bringing to light the intertwining connections between race, poverty, health, and medicine. While the primary factor of poor health was poverty, it was not the only one, as Edward Beardsley has pointed out. Economic factors and housing, schools, nutrition, sanitation, and for African Americans, racism and segregation were all interconnected contributors to the health status in the South affecting health care delivery.[5] As the scholars of the history of medicine Susan M. Reverby and David Rosen argue, to flesh out these connections one must explore not just people of color but the "concept of race itself as an indicator of power relationships and an underlying assumption inherent in medical thinking."[6] Recent scholarship underscores the complex knitting together of racism and medical authority and illuminates a dynamic process in which they interact and shape each other.[7] As the goal of medicine and public health is to protect people individually and collectively, the dynamic interplay and exchange between Florida's public health nurses, black and white, reveal the "biomedical racialization" in public health policy and practice, particularly in the different ways the public health nurses were both physical and conceptual bridges.[8]

As bridges or intermediaries, the public health nurses were in unique positions to facilitate the flow of policies and data up and down the hierarchical network. This flow showed how beliefs, values, and ideas informed the public health nurses' work and determined people's experience of public health.

Working from the middle of their particular societies, they linked state and national public health policies, nursing and medical proceedings, doctors, midwives, town officials, business leaders, and others in the various communities. Often the only ones positioned to improve the health of those left out of modern medical care, they tapped into any resource that would further their cause to bring health education and health reform to Florida's diverse communities.

There was no equivalence, however, to the "middleness" roles of the black and white nurses. White public health nurses were generally positioned as bearers of middle-class values. They were acculturated and indoctrinated with what historians of the Progressive Era have pointed out was cultural and professional arrogance.[9] Black public health nurses, on the other hand, had much in common with other black women whom Patricia Hill Collins argues were marginalized in society but drew strength from their distinctive Afrocentric women's culture and resisted their economic and political subordination. This "outsiders-within" concept aptly relates to the black public health nurses. On one level they could see the locus of power in the white health facilities, institutions, and nursing associations but on another level understood they remained on the outside, sidelined, exploited, and most commonly earning a lesser wage than their white counterparts.[10] The outsiders-within concept offers a framework to help understand the black public health nurses' agency. Though their focus was on the African American communities, Rosa Williams Brown and others showed how they did not confine their networks to the African American communities to achieve their aims. For both races, the nurses' interactions within the communities underscored real and dynamic relations of racialized power.

Of course, from the "middle out" the white nurses had more opportunities to interact with businessmen, doctors, clubwomen, and city leaders and to encourage a two-way discourse concerning the most optimal way to reach people. People in power, in contemporary terms often referred to as the "best" white people of the community, facilitated—or sometimes obstructed—the public health nurses' messaging about populations left out of modern medicine. Their interactions highlight the problematic nature of implementing northern health initiatives into Florida; they revealed that the state had much in common with its southern neighbors that upheld white supremacist state and local governments and medical establishments.

One of the first to discuss the color-line problematic that so concerned

Reid was the public health nurse leader Mary Sewell Gardner (1871–1961), who wrote a text targeted to public health nurses. In 1938 Gardner updated and published the third edition of her classic *Public Health Nursing*, a manual for public health nurses. In it she discussed what Karen Buhler-Wilkinson describes as "the Southern Dilemma."[11] Gardner cautioned northern nurses to be mindful of the culture where race and class had a profound effect upon the way a public health nurse could deliver her message. "A Northern nurse working in the South will accomplish nothing by ignoring the question of color," Gardner warned. "Many an otherwise good nurse has failed because of her inability to understand conditions new to her." Gardener advised nurses to adapt their work to the local areas. They "need not give up [their] point of view, but may so present it, and so adapt it and so make a good working basis on which [they] . . . may proceed."[12] In Charleston, South Carolina, for example, public health nurses had to face obstructions from many white southerners who were unwilling to support a nursing service that would be tasked with the obligation to care for the health of the black population.[13] Whether in Richmond, Virginia, or other southern cities including those in Florida, the difficulty of sustaining health initiatives in the black population was an uphill battle, even as many white nurses willingly crossed the color line.[14] The interracial nature of their work adds another element to what Elna Green has described as a "quiet world of southern women's interracial activism."[15]

From North to South, Taking Public Health Nursing to Florida

Arriving in the early 1920s, Reid found Florida backward in its public health initiatives as compared to the progressive North. Reid had commanded a leadership position within the US Public Health Nursing Service from the time it was formed in 1919; she accumulated vast experience in Washington DC, the West, and the South. She was in a position to access the late development of the South's state and local health departments and their problems with poor funding, less authority, and a lack of professionally trained staff, including public health nurses.[16] Arriving almost a decade earlier than Reid, Brown also was in a position to compare the South with the North. For Brown, the neglect of black Floridians' health stood out. Before her arrival in Florida, she lived and worked in New York, the hub of public health nursing activities. Soon after her 1907 graduation from Lincoln Hospital Training School for Nurses in New York, she secured a position as the head nurse in the city's Colored Orphans

Asylum in the Bronx and observed the growing demand for and organization of visiting nurses within the city. She did more than observe, however. Joining with Adah Thoms and other black nursing leaders, Brown was a founding member of the National Association of Colored Graduate Nurses, an organization established in 1908 to strengthen and professionalize the education and work of black nurses. The fledgling organization required the ammunition Brown provided from her fact-finding tour in the South.[17]

Brown's investigations and reports on work done by the "colored nurses in America" placed a great emphasis on the accomplishments of the sparse numbers of visiting nurses she encountered. "Prevention of suffering is as much her work as nursing," she stressed. Yet she could assess how much more could be accomplished with the cooperation and organization present in northern states. "The negro nurse in New York city, Pennsylvania, and other northern states is taking her share of this social movement but she, unlike the nurse in the south, has the advantages in the organized and systematized work for which she receives remuneration," she charged. Brown argued that the deficit impeded the black professional nurses' work in the South, a shortfall that would include Florida.[18] On one level, therefore, in this book I explore Brown's agency and that of her counterparts in their uphill struggle to make inroads into nurses' professional development and the subsequent delivery of specialized care.

On another level, I examine how the nurses, black or white and whether educated in the North, West, or South, brought public health initiatives that stemmed from the North into Florida. Laurie Jean Reid believed it was she who led the way, declaring in 1922 that the status quo in Florida was so far removed from the North that a public health nurse must arm herself with a "professional training and the pioneer spirit" to muster the "courage to blaze the trail for better living conditions for those who shall come after." While the nurses "ought to have permanent place in every county and community," Reid conceded such aims were a long way off.[19] Reid and Brown based their assessments on the exponential growth of organized public health nursing work in the North during the first two decades of the twentieth century.

In the late nineteenth century, Lillian Wald (1867–1940) and Mary Brewster (1864–1901) of the Henry Street Settlement House in New York initiated the ground-breaking nursing programs to address the social and medical needs of the poor immigrant communities of the Lower East Side. Visiting nurses, the forerunners of public health nurses, fanned out from Henry Street and within a decade expanded their work to include other neighborhoods across the city including Harlem.[20] Tuberculosis nursing, school nursing, and infant welfare were incorporated into the work and became pilot programs for expanded work.[21] The goal of school nursing, for example, was to protect children in school from contagious diseases, supplement the medical inspections, and teach children the principles of good health. In the initial Henry Street nursing service, nurses followed up on children's ailments by visiting them in their homes; the service resulted in an increase in school attendance. Thus, school nursing took root in New York with the municipal employment of the first twelve nurses and provided a model that spread from city to city.[22]

Most public health nursing programs began in the Northeast and spread to the West and the South. By 1912 public health nurses were employed by public and private funds, and the field had expanded to include work for insurance policy holders, schools, factories, department stores, hotels, tenements, small holdings, cities, towns, and some rural areas.[23] The success of the nursing programs on a local level had stimulated Wald to push for reforms on all issues affecting children in a move that involved the national government. She proposed a children's bureau and facilitated its introduction to Congress in 1906. At the time of the first White House Conference on Children's Health in 1909, President Theodore Roosevelt endorsed the proposal; on April 19, 1912, President William Howard Taft signed the founding of the United States Children's Bureau into law.[24] Subsequently, the Children's Bureau significantly cleared the nurse's road to public work. Under the leadership of Julia Lanthrop, the first female head of a federal agency, the Children's Bureau provided leadership on a national level to address all matters concerning the health and welfare of the nation's children and pave the way for the implementation of the Sheppard-Towner Maternity and Infancy Protection Act—and Reid's arrival in Florida.[25]

In Florida, as elsewhere, public health nurses traveled long distances, often alone, to reach neglected populations. Their work, therefore, demanded an authority that they drew from their professional identity. Henry Street nurses set the bar. Professionalization was contingent upon the provision of nurses who had graduated from credentialed nursing schools. Lillian Wald coined the term "public health nurse" in 1912 to identify those who graduated from accredited nursing schools and worked in the public realm to reach people in their homes. She believed a public health nurse would answer "every call for help, without regard to race or creed or religion."[26] To develop this road into public life and unite the nurses in their common goal, Wald,

Gardner, Jane A. Delano (1862–1919), and others formed the National Organization for Public Health Nursing.[27] The nursing organization was the only one of the era that accepted black nurses as well as lay membership. The inclusion of black nurses was not surprising since they were employed in the Henry Street Settlement House, paid equal salaries, and accorded professional courtesies and recognition. Yet as Darlene Clark Hine points out, black nurses were not sent to white homes or promoted to supervisory positions, a policy that reflected deep-rooted racism present in the North as well as the South.[28] While the national leaders encouraged public health nurses to become activists and inform national and local public health policy, racism compounded their difficulties.[29]

The founding of the Red Cross Rural Nursing Service in 1912 marked the establishment of the third important national organization that year to support the progress of public health nursing nationally; it led to eventual consequences for Florida. It was Wald who drove the idea of expanding the nurses' work from urban to rural areas and the visionary Jane Delano who channeled the American Red Cross toward public health nursing.[30] Moving from national leadership into local communities, the promising start to the American Red Cross rural public health nursing expanded into the Red Cross Town and Country Service, offering opportunities for Red Cross public health nurses to find work in the South. They did not reach as far south as Florida.[31] Still, the Red Cross began to influence health care in Florida in a different way.

Through a nationwide partnership with community leaders the Red Cross developed innovative ways to fund the fight against tuberculosis. Florida's clubwomen wholeheartedly participated and went on to back the subsequent employment of local public health nurses to fight the devastating disease commonly dubbed "the white plague." After World War I, the Red Cross nursing service took further steps in Florida to influence the development of public health nursing in the state, and in doing so it added a layer of complication to Reid's leadership.

Creating Career Paths in Black and White

Florida's first public health nurses belonged to a new group of career women forging a profession that came of age in the Progressive Era, but attitudes among national, regional, and state nursing leaders created a wide variance of opportunities for white and black graduate nurses. Throughout the country, in the North as well as the South, the material practice of racism informed the nursing profession including Red Cross nursing developments. The process of working toward their professionalization therefore was complicated by race.

National nursing organizations founded by dynamic nurse leaders were critical to setting standards and goals for the new profession. The National Association of Colored Graduate Nurses was formed more than a decade later than the national association for white nurses. Founded in 1896, the Nurses Associated Alumnae changed its name in 1911 to the American Nurses Association. The organization reflected racial bias. The prominent nurse leader Lavinia Dock, secretary of the International Council of Nurses, invited Brown to represent the Association of Colored Graduate Nurses at the International Council of Nurses convention in Cologne, Germany, in 1912. For Dock, the racial discrimination within the American Nurses Association was a "cruel" and "destructive" practice. She urged fellow nurses to embrace a more inclusive policy: "I do hope that in this one human problem, in dealing with the question of the negro race in America, that there, especially, we nurses will exercise and simply practice that one simple rule, to treat them as we would like to be treated ourselves."[32] Her words, however, were not heeded; regardless of Jim Crow laws, daughter state associations followed the parent organization's lead in excluding black graduate nurses.

In Florida, white graduate nurses organized a local body in Jacksonville in 1909. Three years later, driven by some of the State Board of Health's first nurses, the State Graduate Nurses Association of Florida was formed to serve the white graduate nurses of the whole state.[33] The founding of the association lagged behind that of many in the North and the South, illustrating the tenuous nature of a profession in its infancy.[34] In spite of Brown and other black nursing leaders' efforts, black nurses did not formally organize in Florida until 1935, trailing the professionalization of white nursing even further. Later, however, Florida played a key role in the integration of the national organizations.[35] Not surprisingly, throughout the Jim Crow era, white graduate nurses were a more visible presence in Florida as they developed their profession and worked in the public health arena.

As in the rest of the South and the nation, black graduate nurses were faced with an "outsiders-within" perception and forced to recognize—even as they resisted—that their careers were limited because of their race. Though the major thrust to establish the public health nursing profession in Florida during the first half of the 20th century fell upon the white professional nurses, the black professional nurses certainly were not passive participants.[36] Black nurses struggled to advance their careers with Florida's leaders seated firmly at the center stage of the national movement. These leaders bring Florida's lesser-known black women to light and show how they became health activists and nursing organizers with a primary goal: to save lives and improve health in the African American communities of Florida.

The Backdrop to the Public Health Nurses' Work in Florida

In the following pages I set the stage for the first public health nurses to begin work for the State Board of Health in 1914. The fight against tuberculosis— the white plague—drew the first three public health nurses of the State Board of Health to travel the state, reach out to the rural areas, and initiate contact in neglected black communities. These nurses provide a lens to explore the importance of Florida's geographic construction, climate, and settlement patterns and to highlight the interconnections of race and class with public health, medicine, nursing, disease, and women's place in Floridian society. By 1916, when the number of public health nurses increased to thirteen, their work had expanded to include other diseases and health concerns that grew out of Florida's climate, environment, and poverty. The nurses underscore the consequences of a marriage between racialized medicalization and the state's public health policies that began in 1889 with the creation of the State Board of Health.

While Florida's particular geographical location and physical environment accentuated the challenges of the public health nurses' work, those conditions also contributed to the necessity of establishing the State Board of Health in the first place. In the late nineteenth century, busy port cities strategically located on the east and west coasts of the peninsula were open for trade with other states, the Caribbean, and the rest of the world. Jacksonville, in the northeast corner of the state, Pensacola on the west coast in the Panhandle, and Key West at the south end of the Keys were the largest cities and thriving ports, followed by Tampa and St. Augustine. Land-locked Tallahassee was chosen the state capital for its location midway between Pensacola and Jacksonville. In a state with 1,200 miles of coastline, the port cities and smaller coastal towns were particularly susceptible to the virulent yellow fever epidemics of the late nineteenth century.

Of the many yellow fever epidemics in the South, in 1888 Jacksonville suffered the worst, with 4,656 cases.[37] The high death toll, paired with the crippling disruption to the city's commerce, forced a special session of the state legislature to establish the State Board of Health on February 20, 1889. It was the first official governmental step toward a state public health system. Florida was a laggard in establishing this important milestone as compared to other southern states. Southern leaders in public health considered the move overdue. They claimed that if Florida already had a state board in place, as did South Carolina, Louisiana, and Tennessee, "instead of the medley of competing, inefficient county boards," the Jacksonville epidemic would have been contained.[38]

In his first official act as governor, Francis P. Fleming signed the law creating the State Board of Health in name and function. The three-person official policy-making board made up of "discreet citizens" in turn appointed Dr. Joseph Y. Porter (1847–1926) as the first state health officer. The board became an entity headquartered in Jacksonville and led by an all-male cast of white doctors and "discreet citizens" with certain powers to enforce laws. Porter was an officer with the US Marine Hospital Service in Key West and heralded for his tireless effort to control Jacksonville's yellow fever epidemic. He immediately set about advancing methods of quarantine and fumigation to avert future outbreaks of yellow fever brought into the state.[39]

During his tenure in Florida lasting for twenty-eight years, Porter witnessed enormous strides in medical advances that changed the nature of diseases. In 1905, by the time the last yellow fever epidemic occurred in Pensacola, the etiology of the disease was well understood and the outbreak quickly contained. As some measures became obsolete, however, Porter continually struggled with the legislature to update laws and provide adequate funding to support public health necessities such as steps to improve the reporting of vital statistics. The continual want of funds foreshadowed the difficulty of eventually including nurses as a part of the public health team alongside physicians and other citizens. For the first twenty-five years of the board's existence, Porter relied solely upon doctors and reform-minded citizens to institute and support measures to control epidemics, avert infectious diseases, and promote environmental sanitation.[40]

Florida was no exception to the larger picture of public health problems that were found throughout the country and stemmed from conflict between individual liberty and the government's attempts to impose health regulations to protect the welfare of the larger community.[41] People demanded protection for their individual rights that was further complicated in Florida as in the rest of the South, where the states and counties were more concerned with their own localities and issues of class, kinship, and religion than a state-imposed, broad social welfare policy. Porter took issue with such self-serving attitudes. It was especially galling to him when he had devised ways to educate the public and lay out health updates and news concerning the statewide function of the State Board of Health in local newspapers and a specially produced monthly public health magazine *Florida Health Notes*. He believed the publication would "stimulate an interest in sanitary matters, not only in the masses, but arouse those who are charged with the protection of the public health in the counties to active measures." Yet, many still were reluctant to endorse state health measures at the expense of their personal lives. Toward those citizens Porter unleashed his wrath, complaining that they looked at health officials as "interlopers and principally desirous of asserting a czarism . . . which many in the community contend as unnecessary in interference with commerce or travel."[42]

In fact, Porter went further and in 1907 argued that in his experience one might expect that opposition to public health measures would come from the "ignorant and poorer class of citizenship, for usually ignorance and poverty go hand in hand." However, it was more likely the "wealthy citizens who start the cry of tyranny by the health authorities." Porter contended that even though more wealthy citizens were targeted with newspapers and *Florida Health Notes*, they "provoked hostility when their comfort, pleasure or business was interrupted."[43] He simply did not have the legislative backing to impose policies that some might see as coercive, such as compulsory smallpox vaccination. As William A. Link points out, many southerners' conception of personal liberty had consequences, as "localism worked against progressivism."[44] By filling a space between localism and progressivism, the public health nurse could connect health policy to reach those left out of modern medical care. To facilitate their work they needed to induce recalcitrant citizens to comply. It was an uphill battle. Often they had to enlist help from uncooperative doctors, as one nurse in 1916 reported: "If they [physicians] would only keep their addresses and names, so I could find them for it is the negro and ignorant white people that we especially wish to locate."[45]

During Porter's tenure Florida's population base was both static and changing. Living in the more static rural areas were many of those Porter considered the "poorer class of citizenship" who were simply out of reach to provide challenges to his authority. Black and white poverty-stricken tenant farmers and laborers of the Panhandle and the north central counties eked out livings in an agricultural and lumber economy. Many of the rural dwellers relied on their own cures, medicines, and childbirth practices. Some were former slaves and their descendants who, like George Pretty, came to Florida in 1893 from Pennsylvania to farm near Palatka. He knew all the roots and herbs and was "often found gathering and using them upon his friends and neighbors."[46] Others were like the ninety-year-old sharecropper Rebecca Hooks. From her home in Lake City she told of midwives who had been more popular than root doctors on plantations and brewed medicine for every ailment. They handed down their skills to Hooks and her counterparts.[47] Still others like Bolden Hall and Charlotte Mitchell Martin relocated from Florida's slaveholding plantations to Live Oak. Martin practiced "herb doctoring," and she reported to the interviewer that "doctors sought her out when they were stumped on difficult cases."[48] Though brief, Martin's note adds a layer of complexity to the midwifery story in Florida.

In the 1890s the rural areas were home to approximately 80 per cent of the population of Florida, and although herb doctoring lessened, home births remained common practices into the waning years of Jim Crow. The public health nurse Jule O. Graves (1881–1961), who arrived at Florida's State Board of Health in 1926, snapped photographs and recorded snippets of stories of the lives of many of the rural people living during Porter's tenure. Not all the midwives were black or female; some were male, both black and white. Graves wrote of one unidentified white male midwife, for example, who hailed from Georgia, where he began delivering babies in 1894. "Learned to do deliveries on a stock farm delivering hogs," Graves scribbled in a note on the back of his photograph. "Delivered his first human mother young colored mother in the back of a wagon."[49] By 1930, when the board's program to educate midwives was in full swing, the rural population remained a significant figure even though it had dropped to 50 percent and included rural dwellers of other areas around Lake Okeechobee and South Florida. By 1960 the rural population had declined yet again, to 26 percent. From 1914 to 1964, the people living in these rural areas became an important focus for the public health nurses. Many black women continued to embrace the services of midwives whether by choice or necessity in rural and urban areas.

But as the retired black public health nurse Grace Higgs (1910–1998) pointed out, during Jim Crow, while most white mothers were heading to hospital for their deliveries, it was primarily overarching institutionalized racism that in-

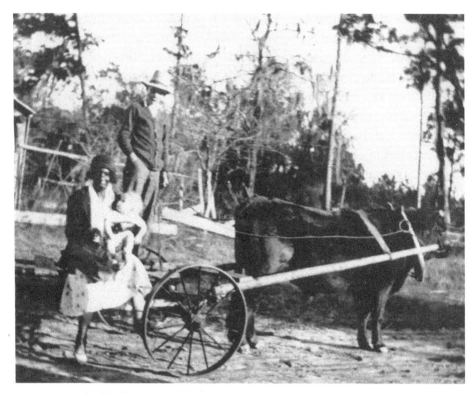

Figure I.2. A midwife holding a small child sits in an ox-drawn wagon in rural Florida, ca. 1930. Courtesy of the State Library of Florida.

formed a black woman's decision to engage a midwife. "Black women had a hard time getting into hospital . . . and [the hospital] would only take [mothers] if they had complications," she recalled. "That's where the midwives served their purpose. It was not a matter of who didn't want to go [to a hospital], it was a matter that they just weren't accepted."[50] Higgs's reflection enhances an understanding of midwifery when the board's midwifery program expanded in the 1930s. It illuminates the importance of utilizing oral histories as valuable tools for historical reconstruction.[51] Oral histories and memoirs help to examine points of connection, tension, or alienation and deepen an understanding of the consequences of the social construction of health.

During the first decades of the State Board of Health's existence the rural areas remained culturally static, while new modes of transportation opened South Florida to welcome residents often hailing from the North, the Midwest, the Caribbean Islands, and northern parts of Florida. In the 1890s the north Florida markets depended on rail transportation that required rail lines traversing from east to west and south as far as Tampa. Access to the port cities and railway terminals was limited to country roads suitable for horse-drawn carts and carriages. Most of south Florida was swampland. There was no Palm Beach, Fort Lauderdale, or Miami as we know them until Henry Flagler's trains opened up the southeast coast in 1896. The train tracks continued south to connect the Florida Keys and in 1912 arrived in Key West. By then destructive freezes had moved the citrus industry south, and speculators had begun to drain the great swampland south of Lake Okeechobee to make way for the building boom.[52] An increase of automobiles and better roads were factors that fed Florida's great land boom of the 1920s. Access to an automobile as early as 1914 and travel on better roads certainly facilitated the public health nurses' travel to rural areas. Road building was a function of local government, but after 1924 the state took responsibility for the statewide construction of highways. In 1924, 749 miles of new highways were completed and by 1930, 3,254 miles.[53] Still, as one public health nurse noted when she started work in 1930, the roads remained a problem. She learned to "drive a Model A Ford where there were no roads, to keep in the ruts in the sand roads, to drive through streams, as there were few bridges, and if there was a bridge to stay on the good planks."[54]

The opening of south Florida drew people of both races, although the majority of the new residents were white and headed to the counties along the east and west coasts. When the State Board of Health began operation, however, approximately 40 percent of the state's population was African American, a figure that remained static between 1890 and 1915 even as the population soared from 400,000 to almost a million. After World War I and by 1920 the Great Migration to the North decreased Florida's black population to 34 per cent. By 1960, when the total population had risen to five million, the African American ratio had dropped yet again, to 26 percent.[55] Those who remained in Florida during the Jim Crow era were subjected to the customs and laws of the South that separated the races socially and politically.

Florida led the way in 1887 by passing a series of Jim Crow laws intended to subjugate African Americans socially.[56] They began with the railroad law, separating races when traveling by train, and later extended to include streetcars, taxis, hotels, restaurants, and hospitals. In 1890 poll taxes subjugated African Americans politically as well. The 1896 US Supreme Court decision in *Plessy v. Ferguson* justified segregation in the "separate but equal" ruling and reinforced such subjugation.[57] The new towns of Florida embraced segregation, following the pattern of the older ones throughout the rest of the South. Historians of racialized medicalization in the South have shown the consequences of this policy that resulted in poverty, overcrowding, and poor sanitation and contributed to the morbidity and mortality rates among African American residents.[58] In Florida, too, whether African Americans lived in cities or rural areas, they were relegated to the bottom rungs of the economic ladder, where they faced material deprivation including an absence of medical care.[59]

In young Miami, city planners relegated the African American community to the bleakest part of town, dubbed "Colored Town." In 1908 city fathers were alerted to an unnamed illness erupting in Colored Town and feared that an epidemic would break out. Upon their visit to this segregated part of town they "found things were in a deplorable condition." The decision to avert an epidemic, however, was an easy one! First patch up the ill people in a makeshift tent and then send them away from the burgeoning new city—out of sight and reach. The city fathers simply appealed to Flagler's Florida East Coast Railway for passes "to get these people free passage from whence they came."[60] This was indeed a magic spell cast by the "Magic City" to make seemingly undesirable residents disappear. Neither the well-being of these African American victims of disease nor their deplorable living conditions were worthy of consideration. It was an example of what Samuel Kelton Roberts describes as "infectious fear" that bore consequences. The United States Public Health Service physician Carroll Fox, who evaluated Florida's State Board of Health in 1915 spelled out one ramification. He blamed the African American people themselves for the problems of sanitation that caused the outbreak of disease. He declared the sheer number of African Americans living in the state "was the reason the problems in sanitation became more difficult to solve."[61] Race motivated medical thinking. Such thought in public health practice set the tone for the public health nurses' work as well.[62]

Throughout the Progressive Era most white medical authorities justified the cause of problems with black health on biological "inferiority," a term that spoke to the medicalization of racism.[63] The mortality rate for African Americans was almost twice that of whites, leading many to conclude that the cause stemmed from the inferiority of the black race that according to white supremacists would surely lead to its extinction.[64] Many of the white supremacists were influenced by a new breed of "scientific" historians led by a Johns

Hopkins professor, Herbert Baxter Adams, who drew on the Teutonic germ theory to claim that the ability for self-government could only pass through the white race's "pure blood lines." This view suggested that slavery was a positive force that did not prepare blacks for political equality but for second-class status.[65] In its seemingly scientific language the basis of the Teutonic germ theory gave credence to a broader pattern of white power, adding weight to authority, abuse, and neglect.[66]

Scientific advances of the era based on the discovery of microorganisms, however, forwarded another type of germ theory that did not recognize the color line and had a profound effect on the development of public health practice and people's lives. Scientific proof for the germ theory of disease provided by Joseph Lister, Louis Pasteur, Robert Koch, and others precipitated the bacteriological revolution, and by 1900 it was widely accepted by the medical and public health profession. To be sure, improvement in public health depended not only on the science but also on the social factors such as the elevation of the standard of living and positive community response and reinforcement to reform measures.[67] Improving living standards for Florida's out-of-reach population was a public health aim and one of the public health nurses' goals. If advances in microbiology and the development of the germ theory led to a gradual improvement of black health, though, the germ theory also heightened scientific racism.[68]

The incident in Miami illustrated a consequence of scientific racism, and Jacksonville's City Health Officer Charles E. Terry (1878–1945) supplied another. Both outcomes provide background to the public health nurses' deployment of health policy. The historian James Crooks credits Terry for his schooling in progressive medical practices. He was a "new breed of urban reformer . . . laying the foundations for contemporary health practice."[69] Terry was in line with others in Baltimore and elsewhere who built a foundation with the premise that public health authorities take at least modest responsibility for all citizens—but without a consideration of what that citizenship meant.[70] He justified his concern for the high mortality rates in the African American community with a blunt condemnation of racial mixing. "We must pay the penalty of race infection," he argued, "people are so intermingled in our lives, in the kitchen, the nursery, our stores and factories carrying to our food and babies their own infections that, regardless of all unselfish motives, we cannot but recognize their danger to ourselves and should use all effort to guard them from their ignorance."[71] Missing from his dialogue was an understanding of the social and economic context and in fact the interdependence between races. His recourse was to present comparative statistics of the large mortality rate among the city's black citizens as compared to the white race to the attention of Jacksonville's African American leaders. In 1911 there were 107 black stillbirths compared to 35 white ones.[72] It was therefore not state or city funds that supported the first black city health nurse but rather philanthropic black leaders who created the Colored Health Improvement Association of Jacksonville and raised funds to support this nurse's initial employment. The medical historian David McBride points out that within the black community a voluntary public health movement emerged to address its own health needs.[73] Such community action underscores Rosa Williams Brown's point that a black public health nurse "could see the needs of . . . our people as no one else could."[74]

According to the evaluator Fox, in 1915 Jacksonville and Miami were the only cities in Florida with health departments "worthy of the name." The employment by the state of black and white public health nurses was critical to cover vast areas of unserved territory.[75] The board's willingness to advocate for state funds to employ a black nurse was in response to Fox's suggestion. In yet another example of scientific racism he advised the appointment by clarifying that "some colored nurses" would help to "prevent the spread of disease to the white population . . . and conserve the life and health of the laboring class of the South."[76] The hiring of a lone black nurse was typical of the state's inadequate response to address black residents' health, a neglect that was reflected throughout the South, but it was at least a start. Yet, there were more clouds over the board's positive if small step. The weight of the eugenic philosophy took hold nationally in the public health realm, influencing policy and thereby some of the well-trained public health nurses like Laurie Jean Reid as well.[77]

The short-lived first public health nursing service of the board provided a springboard to examine how theories of race and disease played out between the nurses, Florida's neighborhoods, and the lonely frontier. After Porter's tenure and as the Progressive Era waned, new studies in physiology, genetics, and anthropology fed into the specialized fields in medicine, public health, and sociology-anthropology. When the poor health of servicemen during World War I alerted the nation to the health crisis among blacks, the medical authorities and philanthropists sought to address the African American population's health more vigorously.[78] New theories emerged explaining black-white differences in health outcomes. While it demarked the races by accepting physical and genetic characteristics, it recognized that both black and white people had similarities in common, namely inborn immunities and susceptibilities to disease. Medical authorities expected to administer treatments with positive outcomes to all, regardless of race.[79] The public health nurses' continuing mission drove them to connect such medical treatments to two groups of people in particular, the rural and the African American poor living in Florida.

Rooting a Woman's Dominion and Promoting a New Profession

The public health nurses' need to discover, alleviate, and prevent suffering, particularly among the poor who suffered from tuberculosis, was first brought to the fore by Florida's forward-thinking clubwomen. In the first decade of his tenure, Porter wrote in *Florida Health Notes* about the "fight for cleanliness" in homes and cities, the value of fresh air, sunshine, and good nutrition, and precautions to be observed when people with infectious tuberculosis descended upon the state.[80] In the second decade of his tenure he learned that one of the most effective ways to implement preventive measures to avoid disease in public spaces was for women to take the antituberculosis message into their communities and people's homes.

Florida's gentle winters had long drawn people seeking to improve their health. Many were drawn by promoters like Harriet Beecher Stowe, who wrote to her northern readers in 1873 that "consumptives and all other invalids" would benefit from a winter in Florida.[81] Others followed advertisers like the surveyor and developer of Orange County, John A. MacDonald, who traveled south as an invalid. "I was alarmed at the condition of my lungs," he wrote in a promotional leaflet urging others to head to the undeveloped southern parts, where the health and prosperity that Florida could offer awaited their arrival.[82] Scores of invalids sought sanctuary in the country's southernmost state, causing many in Florida's medical community to attribute the growing problem of the white plague to the "damyankees" who brought it from the North.[83]

"Your son has consumption. His case is hopeless" were certainly "words to freeze the soul" that medicinal advertisements used to capitalize on people's fear of the disease.[84] People spoke of tuberculosis in hushed tones, often preferring euphemisms in obituaries.[85] The practice added a layer of complexity to the reporting of accurate death statistics. It was not until the opening of the state laboratory in 1903 that Porter had a clearer estimate of deaths caused by tuberculosis—a startling 742, but the count was undoubtedly higher.[86] The state legislature did not provide funding to allow for the collection of vital statistics.[87]

Porter's impending struggle with the legislature over how best to fund the treatment of tuberculosis played out in significant ways. He believed isolation was the answer to prevent the danger of infection; he proposed to the legislature that the state fund "shack shelters" or "tent towns" away from centers of population where the "sufferers could drink in nature's curative power."[88] The legislature did not respond favorably, and similar requests failed as well. Sanitariums, isolation hospitals, and boarding houses sprang up throughout Florida, but there were no institutions, state, county, or private, that could accommodate the indigent consumptive. In 1909 the legislature finally agreed that the State Board of Health should acquire and maintain a sanitarium for the indigent, but the agreement did not hold. The legislature diverted the money to pay the Confederate pension fund.[89] Meanwhile, Porter discovered a powerful group of women who joined the antituberculosis crusade, endorsed his policies, and found a way to deliver his message to those with and without homes.

This group of women, a mix of clubwomen, doctors, and professional nurses, took up the mantle to help disseminate the Progressive Era message for healthy living. The antituberculosis campaign was fertile territory for their outreach. Furthermore, it was the women doctors and clubwomen who demanded legislative backing to support the public health nurses when they first stepped out into communities as tuberculosis nurses. Their determination to get things done was not surprising and reflected goals in common with other Progressive Era women reformers.[90] In one public health nurse's words, Florida's clubwomen were the "power behind the throne. . . . In very many instances are laws passed not from a sense of duty always, but rather to lessen the continued agitation of the Club women."[91]

The public health nurses' rapport with clubwomen began when the first state health nurses prompted them to address the local sanitation laws as well as exert their influence to draw in local doctors to the cause. The public health nurses' professional status allowed them more power than the trained bedside nurses working in the traditional confines of hospitals and under doctors' immediate authority.[92] Their standing in the community allowed for collaboration on a more equal footing with the clubwomen when they worked together for mutual goals. Laurie Jean Reid was relentless in her pursuit of their support for the Sheppard-Towner Act. She spoke at local and state club meetings, wrote for The Florida Clubwoman, and continually updated them on the progress in midwives' education.[93]

The common ground that connected Florida's women—the clubwomen, doctors, and public health nurses—was what Robyn Muncy terms a "female dominion" to suggest the influence women had in their dominance of maternal health and child welfare, but it is also a term that reflects the confines of their authority.[94] If a white female dominion formed a foundation to initiate and support public health nursing in Florida, it too reflected a limited power. This played out in the clubwomen's inability to maintain the continuum of the state's public health nursing program between 1917 and 1922. Still, the bond of the dominion was not jeopardized. During the void of state health nurses, clubwomen actively sought to empower public health nurses locally at the city and county levels.

Alongside the white dominion, health-conscious women in the black communities took up the mantle to improve health. They were inspired by dynamic national leaders who challenged white women to join their cause. One was Mary Church Terrell, the first president of the National Association of Colored Women. In 1899, speaking to an audience of mostly white women at the National Congress of Mothers, she advised that the future well-being of African American children must bring the races together. She urged the audience to do everything in their "power by word and deed" to offer black children the same opportunities as white children "in the name of justice and humanity, in the name of helplessness and innocence of childhood, black childhood as well as white childhood."[95] Her words carried a personal weight. She had borne four children, but three died soon after birth in tragedies she attributed to inferior medical care in a segregated hospital in Washington, DC.[96] In Florida, leadership formed the Florida State Federation of Colored Women's Clubs, established in 1908, and notable activists like Mary McLeod Bethune (1875–1955) who strengthened the organization. Bethune became its fourth president in 1917 and by then had established links with the first state health nurses.[97] Although black nursing schools were established in Florida, it was the National Association of Colored Graduate Nurses that drove the leadership of professional black nursing such as the inspiring Rosa Williams Brown. With different motivations and levels of visibility than the white dominion, these women fought for uplift in their communities. The public health nurses showed that in spite of segregation and discriminatory practices, the shared mission to improve health brought races together in some measure.

In the first two decades of the twentieth century the profession grew unevenly. For that reason the scope of this book proceeds chronologically and laterally, centering on the public health nurses' work and addressing how they

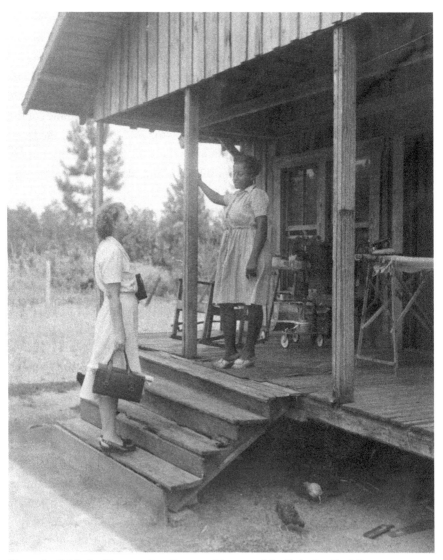

Figure I.3. Public health nurse Ann Preston visits a rural family in Bradford County, ca. 1944. Courtesy of the State Library of Florida.

served those who were out of reach of modern medical care. One of the distinguishing aspects illustrates how and why they got their jobs and opportunities in the first place. Chapter 1 defines the work of the new state nurses as they began to wake up communities in Florida's small towns and the neglected rural communities. Forward-thinking clubwomen paved the way for white pioneer public health nurses. When professionalization offered the nurses a means to make connections in the communities, the board's choice of the nurses becomes a lens to explore the problems of the professionalization of nursing for black and white women. The fledgling program lasted only through the fiscal years from 1914 to 1916, but public health nursing grew locally, sustained in part by the long reach of white and black national philanthropic organizations. The public health nurses' connections with the clubwomen and the black and white national nursing organizations offer contrasting stories of professionalization as the nurses conducted their work to improve health in rural and black communities.

Chapter 2 offers new information to Florida's sparse historical record of the Sheppard-Towner Act program from 1922 to 1929. The 1920s brought federal funds to address mothers' and infants' health against the backdrop of racial unrest, the resurgence of the Ku Klux Klan and great violence, enormous growth in South Florida, catastrophic hurricanes in 1926 and 1928, the collapse of the building boom, and the dawn of the Great Depression.[98] Notably, there were no surviving State Board of Health annual reports from 1923 to 1929. In spite of the lack of the annual reports, however, other records of Laurie Jean Reid's management include many first-person accounts that bring to light the role of the public health nurses, black and white, in their service to the state. The public health nurses who worked in the field to implement the Sheppard-Towner Act were essential to the midwifery program once the federal funds were withdrawn.

The influence of the Red Cross Nursing Service in Florida is the focus of chapter 3 and a subject that scholars have largely overlooked. After World War I, the American Red Cross was promoted to become the "social conscience" of the nation, with central leadership from its Washington, DC, headquarters directing policies and values that guided Red Cross nurses around the world and across the country.[99] Records indicate that many if not most of Florida's graduate nurses belonged to the organization whether or not they served as Red Cross nurses during the war. The chapter traces the Red Cross Nursing Service's links to Florida after 1919, when Red Cross nurses forged new paths into public health particularly to seek out the underserved population. The interconnections with race are seen in the work of African American public health nurses like Katura B. Taylor who emerge from the shadows of history. The aftermath of the 1926 and 1928 hurricanes created further opportunities for the Red Cross to implement a more racially open policy toward the employment of African American nurses, including Rosa Brown. Her valuable insights expose the neglect of rural areas of Palm Beach County and the need for public health nurses in the rural areas as an ongoing mission.

Chapter 4 offers greater depth to the examination of the public health nurses' interplay and interconnections with midwives and country people. Jule Graves was a significant presence during the Sheppard-Towner work and led the midwifery program from 1936 until she retired in 1947. Her first-person accounts are critical to understand the maternity issues facing Florida's rural women before the nurses could intervene and the methods she employed to become a bridge to save mothers' and infants' lives. Graves imparted her skills to a new generation of public health nurses including her colleagues Ethel Kirkland and Lalla Mary Goggans. In black and white, respectively, Kirkland and Goggans offer perspectives that deepen insights into the midwifery program as well as their professional relations. Together, the nurses offer a more complicated history than has been presented previously.

The height of the Depression in 1934 was the eve of a new era for public health nursing. In the process of reorganizing the Division of Public Health Nursing into the Bureau of Public Health Nursing with aid from the Federal Emergency Relief Administration,[100] State Health Officer Henry Hanson reiterated an old plea: "We must have [public health nurses] for the rural communities where doctors will not go."[101] Chapter 5 centers on this new era of public health nursing in the reorganized bureau under the leadership of Florida-born and northern-trained Ruth E. Mettinger (1896–1965). Her prior experience in Florida as a nurse employed through the Sheppard-Towner Act and an American Red Cross public health nurse served her well to lead the bureau through the institution of New Deal programs, the development of county health units, and the aftermath of World War II when new opportunities opened up for black public health nurses in the lead-up to the civil rights movement. Mettinger's history offers a nuanced meaning to her tenure from 1934 until she retired in 1963. For almost three decades she attempted to bring her vision that melded the Red Cross's more racially inclusive philosophy into a nursing practice that would address Florida's future needs.

"We need the vision and the persistence of the well-trained nurse to build a better program," wrote Surgeon General Thomas Parran in 1938.[102] "We must make the greatest *new* effort where the greatest saving in lives can be made."[103] Mettinger represented this "new force—new driving power" to lead nursing efforts to fight Florida's old scourges such as tuberculosis, malaria, hookworm, and pellagra as well as to address syphilis more aggressively. She was responsible for planning and supervising the public health nurses' efforts to battle these diseases through county health departments, once they were established throughout the 1930s and 1940s to better serve the town and rural communities. According to *Florida Health Notes*, the public health nurses would continue to bear the brunt of the battle: "Such state-level programs as venereal disease and tuberculosis control, became county health department responsibilities and public health nurses assumed the major responsibility in bringing these services directly to local citizens in each county."[104] These public health policies, however, were inseparable from racist ideology and professional prejudice. In the waning years of Jim Crow, more black nurses took on public health work, and the racist environment they encountered took a personal toll, as oral histories and other first-person accounts have underscored. Social underpinnings clouded the public health nurses' continuing work as Mettinger urged each one to "seek those who need her the most."[105] To be sure, the public health nurses maintained their unique position as the only ones available to reach those unserved by modern medicine. "Day in and day out," Mettinger noted, the public health nurses of Florida traveled throughout their "district, whether it be a county or a city, working, planning, hoping toward better health conditions."[106] Their work, day in and day out, provides a distinct window into the consequences of the cultural construction of health during the era of Jim Crow.

Finally, this book responds to a theme in Jack E. Davis and Kari Frederickson's edited volume *Making Waves: Florida Female Activists in Twentieth-Century Florida*, a collection of essays addressing a broad selection of Florida's twentieth-century women. These women worked for change and pursued goals in a broad array of fields, from politics to the environment to industrial working conditions to civil rights. In his introduction Davis addresses the fact that many Florida women were left out of national studies because Florida was somehow omitted from the region—either it was too far south geographically or not southern enough culturally.[107] In the present book I seek to help fill the void. The determination and fortitude exemplified by the public health nurses places them firmly parallel with other female activists who made waves and shared a commitment to meet the cultural challenges of Florida. But theirs was a quiet activism in which the nurses went about their work, in Reid's words, without "the waving of banners and the blare of trumpets . . . particularly in Florida where so much of the population is rural."[108] Their quiet approach relegated them to the shadows of history, yet through the work of these nurses not only the southernness of Florida stands out but also its distinctiveness. What follows is the little-known history of Florida's black and white public health nurses, who brought much-needed health measures to rural areas and unserved citizens while also opening a professional path for women and laying the groundwork for the community health nurses who strive for social justice today.

1

‖‖

Waking Up Communities and
Seeking Out the Sick in Town
and Countryside, 1914 to 1917

‖‖

When Rosa L. Williams Brown, a charter member of the National Association of Colored Graduate Nurses, relocated from New York to Jacksonville in 1914, she carried with her a pride in her profession and firm conviction that the black graduate nurse was the ideal person to uplift the health of black communities. She had laid out the association's goals in 1912 during a speech she delivered at the International Council of Nurses held in Cologne, Germany. The founding members, she declared, were motivated to organize by the dire need of people who were living out of reach of modern medical care. "We realize that in this age we need trained negro women to cope with existing conditions among our people," she asserted, "and with this in mind this body of colored graduate nurses met in New York in 1908 to adopt a plan by which, with their united strength, they might help alleviate the ignorance and suffering among their people."[1] She was well aware that progressive work in the South was an uphill climb and fell short in comparison to that of her northern sisters. Organized public health nursing at a state level was not yet in its infancy in Florida, but the inclusion of one black with the white graduate nurses in systemized public health work had begun to take root in Jacksonville. If there was to be change in the black communities of this southernmost state, Brown believed the educated public health nurse must take a part in health reform and as a first step separate herself from the familiar practical nurses. In 1914, the year she was elected president of the association, and now married to Dr. Richard

L. Brown, the pioneering nurse brought the organization's high ideals to Jim Crow Florida. She was well armed to face the challenges ahead: "I am indeed proud to be numbered among this body of noble women, who with all the advantages of higher education have retained that missionary spirit which is so commendable in the sight of God."[2]

Brown found that Jacksonville, the largest city in the state, was home to the State Board of Health headquarters and a thriving City Health Department headed by a reform-minded city health officer, Dr. Charles E. Terry. Since his appointment as the first full-time officer in 1910, he had made remarkable strides to respond to the "onward march of public thought in the matter of preventive medicine" as credited by the state's progressive clubwomen.[3] The Health Committee of the Florida Federation of Women's Clubs took an active role in promoting antituberculosis campaigns and supported Terry to secure health reform ordinances such as milk pasteurization and the construction of privies.[4] When he complained that Jacksonville lagged behind other cities that employed public health nurses to carry the antituberculosis campaign into homes, Jacksonville's clubwomen responded with their financial support. Terry credited the clubwomen for establishing the Associated Charities branch in Jacksonville to become the city's most important private welfare agency.[5] Largely funded through the efforts of the Woman's Club of Jacksonville, in 1911 the organization employed Irene R. Foote (1885–1960) as a visiting nurse to address the indigent cases of tuberculosis.[6]

Foote ranks as one of the leaders in the development of public health nursing in Florida. Born in Wisconsin and a 1906 graduate of the nursing school at Minneapolis City Hospital, she accumulated wide experiences as a visiting nurse for the Minneapolis Associated Charities and as a district nurse in Maine prior to her relocation to Jacksonville. She was in the perfect position to help implement Terry's reforms, ally herself with the city's clubwomen, and promote the professionalization of nursing in Florida. In 1912 she cofounded the white State Graduate Nurses Association of Florida and immediately lobbied for the passage in 1913 of the Nurses Registration Act to ensure that all graduate nurses obtained a Florida license to practice.[7] The goal to separate graduate nurses from the practical nurses who had not graduated from nursing schools echoed Brown's objectives and reflected an important step toward the professionalization of nurses of both races.

Included in Terry's sweeping reforms was his move to regulate midwifery and in doing so open the door for the employment of more public health nurses. According to the State Board of Health, midwives who served women throughout Florida and the South were a "grave evil . . . most of them negro women, who are called upon to attend other women of both races at the birth of their children."[8] Yet in the absence of accurate statistics and death registrations for the rest of Florida and the southern states in general, health authorities could not exactly differentiate between physicians' and midwives' deliveries. Even though midwives were not commonly in attendance in the northern states, the death rates as shown in the federal Children's Bureau statistics of 1913 indicate that deaths of African Americans from all diseases related to pregnancy and confinement were almost double those of whites. Of 100,000 cases, there were 15.2 deaths of white women and 26.1 deaths of black women. Such statistics "picture a very great difference in the standards of care at childbirth in these two groups," the report concludes, "and when all the Southern States are included in the death-registration area the magnitude of the problem will be shown by the death rates."[9] Porter's push for the statewide collection of death statistics finally came to fruition in 1919 when Florida became a nationally recognized death registration jurisdiction.[10] Terry, however, took action based on his own collection of statistics for Jacksonville that reported that a third of the stillbirths were delivered by physicians.[11] Still, just as Susan Smith has pointed out in her study of midwifery in Mississippi, public health officials believed criticism of physicians would be counterproductive. Black midwives were an easier target.[12] Terry bypassed the ongoing issue of substandard physician care to concentrate on educating midwives.

The State Board of Health sidestepped its own inaction to regulate midwifery in spite of regular requests from midwives themselves for certificates or licenses. The midwife Isabelle Maynor, writing from Martin County in 1909, noted that her original license was "burned up," and she requested a replacement. Evidently her first letter was ignored, as she inquired, "Tell me why you fail to send [it]." Dr. Hiram Byrd, an assistant state health officer, was no less confused than many midwives. "There must at some time have been some system of licensing midwives," he wrote to Porter, "for every little while some old midwife writes that she has lost her license or got it burned or otherwise disposed of and wants a duplicate. Do you know what it is, or when or how or anything about it?" Porter replied that possibly some physicians furnished their own certificates to trustworthy midwives, but there had been "certainly no legal enactment. I would not encourage the practice."[13]

By 1914 Porter had reversed his position. The growing field of obstetrics in the United States had prompted a campaign against the midwife that fell into two camps. One group favored the midwives' complete abolishment. The other argued that as a midwife was a "necessary evil," she must be trained and regulated until an adequate number of physicians were properly qualified and sufficient maternity hospitals were established.[14] Porter and Terry fell in with the second camp, asserting that a failure to regulate midwives amounted to "legalizing crime in Florida." Ignoring evidence that physician deliveries were also troubling, they branded all midwives together writing in *Florida Health Notes* that as health standards were raised, "ignorant women, operating without any supervision of legal authority and even the implied sanction of the state, [are] a menace to the mother and the child."[15] The board's complaints directed toward the black midwives were reiterated in Florida's newspapers: "They are a menace through their ignorance and by their direct interference with the laws of nature, by their neglect and often by their superstitious foolishness which in extreme cases results in the senseless rites of voodooism."[16] Terry reported that lockjaw in Jacksonville during 1913 caused seven deaths in ten months among babies who were delivered by midwives in the city. During the same period, there were sixty-seven deaths of children who were attended by midwives from their births to their deaths, exposing the bare fact that there was no other health care available for African American families. None of the children was seen by a physician.[17] The void of health care for black children, along with a new focus on the midwife's education, opened a space for the budding practice of public health nursing.

At first physicians instructed the midwives on measures to safely conduct their practice. Each midwife was required to pass an examination and receive a certificate issued by the City Board of Health. The physician's place as educator, however, was quickly assumed by field nurses, considered by the State Board of Health to be more optimal for their maternal qualities, and with "their infinite patience and tact," they were more able to persuade the midwife and the mother to comply.[18] James Crooks points out that Terry's effective campaign to license Jacksonville's midwives was reflected in the reduced number of midwives practicing in the city. In 1913 there were sixty-four unlicensed midwives in Jacksonville; two years later there were twenty-seven licensed midwives.[19] The City Health Department credited the nurses' work for the lowest infant death rate yet recorded.[20] A few larger cities followed Jacksonville's lead with city ordinances to control midwifery, but the problem of addressing midwives' education would consume public health nurses throughout the 1920s and beyond.[21]

Terry's foresight to initiate the employment of a black public health nurse as a field nurse to reach out to the black midwives was exactly aligned with goals set by the National Association of Colored Graduate Nurses. A colleague of Brown, Margaret A. Allen (b. 1878), accepted the position in Jacksonville. Born in Kentucky and a 1901 graduate of Freedmen's Hospital in Washington, DC, Allen also took a leadership role in the national organization. Allen and Brown attended the fourth annual convention, held in Washington, when members elected Brown as the delegate to attend the International Convention in Germany and Allen as the organization's first vice president. In Florida they once again united for the cause. The Browns opened the small Provident Hospital in 1914, and Rosa began work to organize Florida's African American graduate nurses.[22] Allen had already begun her eight-year tenure at the City Health Department, where her work included instructing midwives, seeking out suspected cases of communicable diseases, and in the absence of a physician beginning the "general oversight of the health of the negro children of the city, especially among the poorer and more ignorant."[23]

In selecting Allen, Terry bypassed possible candidates from the African American graduates of Jacksonville's Brewster Hospital School of Nursing. The hospital was founded to serve the black community and graduated its first class of nurses in 1904, but between 1913, when the state registration law passed, and 1915, only four of a total of sixteen graduates had received their state registrations. It was a cause for concern for Brown and one she would later address with the National Association of Colored Graduate Nurses.[24] Terry sought support from the Colored Health Improvement Association of Jacksonville to employ a "colored nurse, a woman trained in Red Cross methods brought from Washington D.C." The notation of "Red Cross methods" reassured the public she was well trained to assume a position of authority even as it cast a shadow on a missed opportunity for the graduates of Brewster Hospital. Fresh from Washington, Allen made her first task within the community to put her training to work to garner the "aid of interested friends to the cause" and seek out the "poorer and more ignorant."[25] The interested friends of the black community were well aware of the critical importance of her work especially to school-age children. The City Health Department employed two part-time white doctors and two full-time white nurses to address the health of white pupils in white schools, but black pupils in their segregated black schools were simply left out.[26]

African American clubwomen backed Allen's work and united to the cause of uplifting the health of the black community. Since the organization of the Florida State Federation of Colored Women's Clubs began in 1908, its growth depended on visionary women who worked to improve the health of their communities.[27] Jacksonville's Eartha M. M. White (1876–1974), for example, established the Old Folks Rest Home in the city with her mother, Clara English White. In 1904 Mary McLeod Bethune opened a school in Daytona and in 1911 a hospital that began with two beds and soon increased to twenty, with a corresponding nurse training school.[28] By 1914 student nurses had expanded their reach to serve needy people in their homes in the surrounding community.[29] White and McLeod were in attendance during the Colored Women's Club eighth annual session of 1915, held in Tampa, when Allen spoke on the topic of health. She told of her work "as a visiting nurse for the Negroes" in which she averaged twenty to forty visits per day—and was the only one available to bring health intercessions into black neighborhoods.[30] The clubwomen saw that Allen's work could serve as a model for other cities, and their support was certainly necessary, as only Jacksonville and Miami

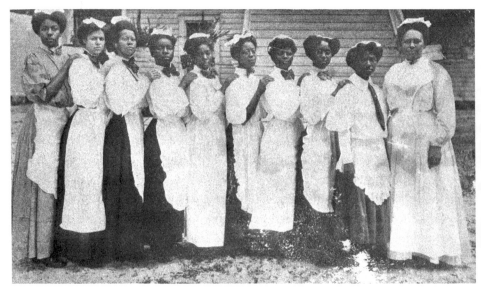

Figure 1.1. The Daytona Literary and Industrial School of Training for Negro Girls offered classes in nurses' training to the senior class, ca. 1911. Courtesy of the State Library of Florida.

supported progressive health departments. If other larger cities of Florida supported local health organizations, they were, in the federal public health evaluator Carroll Fox's estimation, inefficient and ineffective.[31]

Terry's push to obtain a black public health nurse underscored his concern about infant feeding, insect-borne infections, communicable diseases, and the woeful death rate among the African American population. These were matters tied to the underlying social context of racism. While morbidity and mortality statistics informed his assessment of what a black public health nurse could bring to the community, his motive was also based on what he called "self-protection."[32] His reasoning, infused with the pervasive perception that African Americans were disease-ridden due to their biological and moral inferiority, was a recurring theme spelled out for the public in *Florida Health Notes* and often republished as bulletins in local newspapers.[33] "What happens," asked the State Board of Health in *Florida Health Notes*, "when the cook, the nurse-maid, the maid-of-all-work, who live in the quarters or niggertown" arrive to serve white families in their homes? "'Oh! You say, I never go down in niggertown, well perhaps you do not but some of niggertown comes to you."[34] The article stresses that diphtheria, tuberculosis, and any of the communicable diseases could easily be carried from those living in "squalid huts" into white homes. Furthermore, it spelled out the possible consequences of children's interracial play. "How many times have you seen white children playing with the black children in the yards of such houses? . . . [A] white child can contract a fatal case of diphtheria from a mild case in a negro child."[35] While young children of both races commonly played together and learned their social boundaries at an early age, fear of disease simply added fuel to white southerners' rhetoric to separate the races and another layer of reinforcement to the social construction of disease.[36] For action to move forward with his health mission, Terry turned to the philanthropic black leaders who created the Colored Health Improvement Association of Jacksonville and raised funds to support Allen's initial employment. For further action, it was a matter of waking up Florida's communities, a future task for the white and black public health nurses.[37]

Branching Out from Jacksonville

From reforming midwives' education to employing the city's first public health nurses, the progressive initiatives for Florida's health reforms stemmed from Jacksonville, home to the State Board of Health and forward-thinking doctors, professional nurses, and clubwomen. A series of steps initiated by the progressive members of the women's clubs in the antituberculosis fight led to eventual collaboration with the State Board of Health in a major step to extend public health nursing to cover the whole state. The march forward was led by a dynamic woman doctor, Ellen Lowell-Stevens (1864–1945), who arrived from the hub of health progressiveness in New York and in 1906 became the federation's "health chairman." She recognized that the clubwomen were "unprofessional workers," but she understood how best to utilize their strengths.[38]

Lowell-Stevens found that matters of public health, childhood, and education attracted many southern women. Some believed their voices in social reforms would correct male deficiencies, as one woman put it, in "aspects of governmental activity that affected the home."[39] As male politicians appeared indifferent and negligent toward enacting legislation concerning domestic matters, a space opened for women to address them. More generally, reforming clubwomen presumed that women of their class would bring uplift to the community, and thus they pursued a wide range of goals, from public health to child welfare to prohibition. Lowell-Stevens targeted health and led Florida's clubwomen in response to an appeal from the General Federation of Women's Clubs for every federation in the country to appoint a health chairman to join the national crusade against tuberculosis.[40] Lowell-Stevens answered the call to take the "fight against the 'White Plague' . . . into the home" by encouraging clubwomen to focus on their community leadership. Subsequently, Florida's federation provided the public with information by way of educational exhibits and the distribution of literature; it also facilitated the employment of the Irene Foote.[41]

Practical support for the management of tuberculosis control in the state came from the women's clubs directed by Lowell-Stevens and endorsed by the State Board of Health. Demonstrating their successful lobbying powers, clubwomen petitioned Governor Napoleon Broward to appoint Lowell-Stevens as the club's delegate to join Porter at the National Association for the Study and Prevention of Tuberculosis and the Congress on Tuberculosis held in Washington, DC, in 1908.[42] As a result, Lowell-Stevens became aware of the absence but absolute necessity of verifiable statistics in Florida to indicate the extent of tuberculosis in the state. She initiated a grassroots approach by requesting that clubwomen check the deaths in their communities for the previous year. Where there were no town records, clubwomen visited the undertakers to obtain the information. Such lengths indicated the fragile bureaucracy of the State Board of Health. In fact, the first state statistician was not appointed and a Bureau of Statistics was not organized until 1915, a year after the first state health nurses began work.[43] It also indicated the level of collaboration the clubwomen would offer to back the state health nurses when they began to seek out the sick in the clubwomen's home communities. The clubwomen's survey indicated that tuberculosis was prevalent even in the least inhabited parts of Florida.[44] Partly in response to the survey results, Lowell-Stevens again rallied the clubwomen to exert their lobbying power. This time it was to petition the legislature for a state tuberculosis sanitarium.[45] And the clubwomen's powerful lobby prompted the passage of a law in 1909 to provide for one. The legislature failed to follow through with the allocated funds in spite of the clubwomen's continual complaints that the board had deprioritized the sanitarium.[46]

The subsequent dispute between the clubwomen and the board finally came to a head in February 1913. Porter reversed his original desire for a sanitarium, stating that it would do little to solve the tuberculosis problem and the financial consideration was too great. Such a sanitarium to accommodate both races and sexes would become a "charity which Florida taxpayers should not be expected to meet or give," he declared. "If it became known to the States North of us that the State of Florida was maintaining a tuberculosis sanitarium for the indigent," he argued, "this class of individuals would flock down to a warmer climate, and this State would be at an enormous expense in looking after them."[47] Unwilling to budge on the sanitarium issue, Porter recommended that as Florida's climate was conducive to open-air treatment, those suffering from tuberculosis would benefit from isolated outdoor sleeping, rest, and a diet of raw eggs and milk. He maintained that this treatment would be "within the reach of even the poorest."[48] To put the plan in motion, Porter proposed "a corps of trained nurses to travel the State, hunt out the pulmonary consumptive and by advice and continuous assistance, teach . . . the rudiments of healthy living, and thus protect the well members of the family as well as to assist the sick."[49] Florida's clubwomen were dissatisfied with the defeat of their sanitarium campaign and the employment of only three nurses, but in the end Lowell-Stevens conceded that the arrangement was "a beginning at least, even if it did not balance the $30,000.00 to be spent this year on hogs."[50]

The Reunion, the Red Cross, and the Nurse Leader

The legislature's diversion of funds from the tuberculosis sanitarium to supplement property taxes in support of Confederate pensions was, as Elna Green has argued, an underhanded means for the state government to create social welfare programs that supported the Lost Cause movement and reinforced white supremacy.[51] The Lost Cause celebrated what many white southerners saw as the noble fight of the Confederacy to defend their right as sovereign states to make their own decisions. To this end, the South was not defeated, but overcome by the greater numbers of Union military forces. These ideas grew into expressions of celebration in rituals, monuments to honor dead heroes, reenactments, and generous pensions.[52] Even though Florida had become a state that drew northern and foreign residents with opposing views and little tolerance for the Lost Cause, those favoring its intimidating strength drew support from friends in high places and developed one of the most bountiful Confederate welfare programs in the South, a program that continued throughout the Jim Crow era. Significantly, those eligible to receive pensions effectively excluded African Americans, even though the landowners among them paid property taxes to support the pensions. Eligibility rested on Confederate service. Honorable veterans and their widows included poor whites but simply eliminated most blacks.[53]

More overt expressions of white supremacy were expressed in local and regional Confederate reunions; in May 1914 Irene Foote was indirectly involved with the organization of one of the largest reunions in the South, held in Jacksonville. Announcements for the reunion circulated throughout the South with headlines highlighting Florida's generous pension plan to support ex-Confederates. The *Pensacola Journal* reported that Florida promised "a warm and generous welcome" to participants, adding that although Florida was "situated far south of the great theatre of war of 1861–65," the reunion would ease the scar felt from the federal occupation of the city during 1863 and the Union plan to make Jacksonville the "base of operation for the arming of negroes and securing in that way the possession of Florida."[54]

The matter of federal interference and race relations ignited fire at such Confederate reunions. Speakers traditionally condemned the North for abolition, arguing that it threatened "the civilization of the south and the purity of our blood and the integrity of our race." The war was not about the integrity of the union, one insisted, but "simply fought about niggers . . . [W]e fought for the white race in America."[55] To appeal to like-minded people, Florida sold itself as a mecca to keep the Confederate ideology alive: "Florida is not only caring for the living but the memory of the dead is also kept green. Throughout the state handsome Confederate monuments have been erected by both public and private means."[56]

Furthermore, the newspapers expanded on Florida's natural beauty as a selling point to honor the cause, reinforcing the racially charged messages of the South and passing the messages to the next generation. "Florida appeals to the young because of its flowers and its wonders—its poetry, its songs and its attractive history." Its rivers, bays, coastline, and natural vegetation "invest Florida with an interest as wide as the nation."[57] The midwesterner Foote was caught in the middle of celebrations, charged with safeguarding the lives of the aged and infirm veterans, and surely aware of the matter of African Americans' exclusion from white southern society that was left to smolder under the surface.[58]

The sheer volume of 40,000 celebrants descending on Jacksonville prompted the necessity for Foote's nursing supervision of the five Red Cross first aid relief stations. Stretching her professional duties in the city to include early membership of the national American Red Cross Nursing Service, Foote chaired the Red Cross Florida Committee and took charge of relief work during the reunion.[59] The event was without serious medical incident, but Foote was an observer to the hegemony of the Lost Cause. The Red Cross and daily press documented her service but not her voice during the event.[60] Foote's participation reflected her obligation to serve regardless of political undertow, a philosophy drawn from her training and a career path that she carried from the Associated Charities in Minneapolis to Maine and on to Jacksonville.

The outward display of white supremacy in Jacksonville underscored the bedrock of society throughout Florida. For Foote and the first public health nurses the question became whether they could extend their work to negotiate the cultural obstacles and successfully reach out not just to the poor whites but also the African Americans in their homes and workplaces. Foote's answer was to arm herself with additional professional credentials prior to her employment in the field. She was the only state health nurse who attended a public health nursing course at Teacher's College in New York.[61] Clearly, she believed professionalization would strengthen her hand in the community to bring public health work to those living and working in dire health conditions.[62] "I have never been able to refrain from trying to improve conditions that came to my attention," she wrote.[63]

Foote's broader education gave her authority to bring new ideas into Florida. She worked relentlessly to strengthen nursing through the State Graduate Nurses Association, but as African American graduate nurses were denied membership, she recommended a more inclusive stance by organizing the state's Public Health Nursing Association.[64] In Lillian Wald's mold, Foote proposed a state organization that would support all nurses regardless of color. It would also encourage lay membership that in turn would foster support for visiting nursing associations and programs that employed public health nurses.[65] In 1915 Foote's incentive indicated her push to foster broad community collaboration, her drive to improve conditions, and her goal to ultimately save lives. Unfortunately, her effort failed. No records have been preserved.

The First State Health Nurses Start Work

Foote was not among the initial state health nurses in 1914 when the State Board of Health divided Florida into three districts and appointed just three nurses to cover the entire area.[66] Jacksonville, comfortable with its robust City Board of Health, was excluded from the plan. Eula L. Paschall (1880–1958) was in charge of Florida's western district and worked from her hometown base of Pensacola. Harriet J. Sherman (1879–1962) and Frances Herndone (1884–1948) were appointed to the southern and central districts, respectively. Paschall was responsible for seventeen counties, Herndone twenty-four, and Sherman nine. Collectively, they served a rural white and black population of 750,000 spanning a geographical area of 54,861 square miles. Each nurse undertook, as Porter described it in his report, a "hurried general survey tour" to identify "those sections [of the district] in which intensive work should first be attempted." Home visits to tuberculosis patients followed, along with a broad education campaign that encompassed women's clubs, schools, city officials, physicians, boards of trade, and mothers clubs. In their first year the trio visited and treated 207 white and 64 African American patients. Porter recognized the difficulties they faced with delayed rail transportation, poor food in "out of the way places," and crude boarding facilities. Yet despite all the problems of travel, he reported, "They always find the patient, even though it takes a long walk, or drive, or row boat trip combined to reach the destination." Still, he reasoned, it was not reasonable to expect three nurses to accurately survey their districts or meet its needs even if limited to the tuberculosis patient population.[67]

By offering health instruction and advice to people privately in their homes and publicly to the community at large, Porter was satisfied that the state health nurses had shown what could be accomplished with a "full working corps of intelligent women."[68] He was in agreement with Dr. W. E. Bray, a bacteriologist in Mississippi and an expert in rural sanitation who championed the premise of the new profession of public health nursing. Bray contended that rural people were "very religious . . . strong willed and have strong prejudices, and as a class are fond of argument that if they remained healthy as individuals under the old regime, there is no need for new ideas and doctrines." People's deep-seated fatalism regarding illnesses could only be "overcome very tactfully," he noted, making it clear that the public health nurse was the ideal professional to intervene. "Here I think her place is distinctive. She could do many things better than a health officer himself," Bray concluded.[69] Porter recognized that an increase in the nursing force was in Florida's best interest. As state health nurses could "find cases and gain access to homes that can be reached in no other way," their work should extend further than tuberculosis control to cover the many other scourges common to the South and rural areas.[70]

A great strength in supporting an increase in the nursing force came from the state's clubwomen.[71] On November 18, 1914, Porter delivered an address to the clubwomen focusing on the employment of the nurses while also encouraging the women to continue their support of health work.[72] He reiterated that health work connected women in what he described as a "women's part in health work." He specifically pointed out the distinctively womanly province of education in the home. Reinforcing the concept of public housekeeping, he argued, "health is a matter of education; woman is the teacher; home is the school."[73] The clubwomen's concern for the health of the public was perceived by Porter as a natural extension of appropriate female domestic activities and therefore more palatable to many southern men; the clubwomen were creating new roles for themselves no less than the state health nurses were.[74] By underscoring that education was the province of the home, Porter justified the extension of public housekeeping into the homes of rural areas where the terrain was inhospitable, the transportation difficult, and the people possibly hostile. Such challenges required a "capable and self-sacrificing woman" to face and overcome the difficulties, he conceded.[75] Yet he did not acknowledge the importance of hiring professional graduate nurses to become the efficient intermediaries to relay lifesaving measures up and down the hierarchy and into Florida's homes and communities.[76]

Porter framed his argument to the legislature in gendered language. The nurses' outreach required care for both the black and white population, but there was a tacit understanding among legislators that whites came first.[77] Porter argued in terms not of the state health nurses' service to people regardless of color, but on the unique way they served communities. To describe the advantages a skilled state health nurse could bring to family members, Porter drew upon the standard gendered perceptions that women were by their nature sympathetic and that their function as (female) professional nurses was to support the (male) doctors.[78] He stated that the families often preferred talking over problems with a nurse, for the doctor was "always a busy man."[79] Porter did not reveal that nurses were absolutely necessary because doctors often refused to serve indigent or African American patients, as the state health nurses' reports indicate.[80] Taking the lead from the federal Children's Bureau, he pointed out to the legislators that mothers were particularly burdened when tuberculosis afflicted a family's breadwinner. He argued that when household responsibilities fell solely upon a mother's shoulders, frequent visits by a nurse were imperative to ensure that the mother complied with the directions for care. "It can be understood how necessary it is that these unfortunates should be seen frequently in order that their hope may be stimulated and they may observe and fulfill directions for their own care and the protection of their loved ones," he reported.[81] Finally, in line with Bray's conclusion that state health nurses were the ideal professionals to perform the work where often they had to substitute for physicians,[82] Porter was clear in his demand to increase the force. He wrote that the state health nurses have "the wisdom to correct unsanitary conditions, to advise intelligently as to children's diseases and the many ills that commonly occur in rural communities . . . and where services of the physician are not readily and quickly available."[83]

Sensitive to the critical deficit of nursing services, the clubwomen were fully behind the board's move to expand the program. Dr. Grace Whitford (1883–1963), who had taken over as chair of the Florida Federation of Women's Clubs' "Public Health Department," petitioned the legislature for the allocation of additional funds for the nursing positions.[84] In response, in July 1915 the legislature provided funding, allowing the State Board of Health to employ four additional state health nurses. That month, Irene Foote, Mary Spencer, Susan Voorhees (1876–1931), and Lydia Kirk (1874–1957) joined Paschall and Sherman.[85] Nurses were headquartered in Daytona, Gainesville, Jacksonville, Tallahassee, Pensacola, and Tampa; each district encompassed the surrounding six to nine counties. Together they identified an additional 1,225 tuberculosis cases.

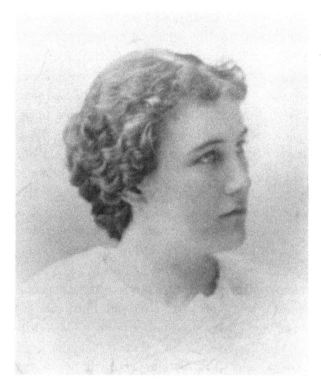

Figure 1.2. Lydia Wheeler Kirk was part of the first graduating class
of Florida's first nursing school at St. Luke's Hospital in Jacksonville,
1895. Courtesy of Gail VanderVoort.

Foote offered the most in-depth reporting of her early work, indicating the
broad span of the nurses' work. Her initial report, highlighted for the public in
Florida Health Notes, illuminated the uniqueness of a service to provide health
care to people regardless of race and one that was essential when there was no
other recourse available. On her first sweep of the east coast district she identified 183 new cases of tuberculosis, among them an eighteen-year-old African
American girl who contracted the disease at a Georgia industrial school. "I
found [the] patient sleeping with a younger sister in a practically closed room,"
she reported. "Both girls were losing in weight had a dry, hacking cough, tired
all of the time, and no appetite." Foote called the family together and instructed
them on a home treatment plan. On her second visit she was "much gratified"
to see the results: "the father had immediately built a sleeping porch on the

second floor, each girl had her own bed, and they were taking from four to six raw eggs and a quart of milk a day apiece. The oldest girl, the first patient, has gained ten pounds and the younger girl six pounds in weight. Neither of these girls could be induced to sleep in the house from now on." The outcome was an exemplar of her own diligence. "This proves the theory that home treatment can be successful if properly carried out with perseverance," she wrote. In be-tween calls to patients, Foote visited doctors, "the mothers club of Key West, the Sans Souci Club of Daytona Beach, the Women's Club of DeLand, [and] the biology class at Daytona High School," teaching them about sanitation, tuberculosis, and the importance of "establishing a local visiting nurse."[86] This grassroots work was critical to the success of the program.

The following year saw the creation of seven more state health nurse ap-pointments and districts, with further headquarters established in Tallahassee, Miami, Lake City, Marianna, Lakeland, and Sanford. Duties expanded to in-clude treatment and education on a range of diseases such as malaria, typhoid, diphtheria, pellagra, pneumonia, and hookworm along with instruction on health care for mothers and infants. The state nursing team embraced the chal-lenges and in December 1916 issued reports to the board detailing the broad expanse of their work.[87] Jessie Wheeler (1872–1958) brought up the hookworm problem, a southern scourge directly related to poor sewage disposal. Florida was the first southern state to launch a hookworm campaign in 1909, but by 1914 the board had pulled back on the initiative, leaving it to local doctors to treat individual cases. As many citizens either failed to access free treatment or were out of reach of local doctors, it was not long before cases of hookworm multiplied. "Some of the toilets in country homes are a disgrace," Wheeler noted, "and there seems to be so much hookworm disease in these sections, though [country people] are very loath to believe that soil pollution causes the spread of this disease."[88] Soil pollution and sewage-borne diseases also caused typhoid fever and dysentery, as Rhea Lee (b. 1888) noted: "Have visited several cases of typhoid fever and pellagra among the poorer classes . . . I of course made a special effort to, and obtained charitable aid" for families in need.[89] Pellagra, yet another southern scourge, was a vitamin-deficiency disease that caused diarrhea, dermatitis, and dementia.

The southern scourges, poor sanitation, and the need to screen outhouses and food stores was a constant theme in many of the reports and an indica-tion of the illness and general health experience of Floridians before they en-countered the traveling nurses. Laura Scott (1874–1944) declared that "people everywhere need waking up to the importance of fresh air and screens."[90] Harriet Sherman found the "sanitary conditions of West Tampa very bad indeed, mostly due to the keeping and stabling of cows in thickly populated parts of town."[91] And Mary Eleanor Roach (1885–1954) echoed that complaint, saying Key West was a "hopeless" case "when a dairy of 26 cows is permitted to exist in the most densely populated part of town."[92] The nurses' grievances about cows stabled in populated areas was a common one; clubwomen all over the South had long campaigned for the removal of cows from city streets, with little success.[93]

Overall, the nurses' reports reveal a distinctively female perspective to health care; the nurses reconciled their professional ideals with goals they shared with the clubwomen whom they looked to for support and collaboration. "In Marion County, the Women's Club labored with me to secure a report from every doctor in the county as to the number and location of tuberculosis cases," wrote Mary Spencer, indicating a power that came with her directive. Irene Foote reported that she "talked before almost every Woman's Club" in her area and asked for clubwomen's assistance "in the matter of stimulating city councils in passing health ordinances, particularly screening outhouses and stores." Susan Voorhees also credited clubwomen for assistance: "Women's Clubs . . . are always ready to respond to any assistance I ask of them in using their influence with city officials in getting things done."[94] Stimulated by the nurses' expanded outreach, the clubwomen became more aware of the dire health conditions affecting both races. "The women of the Federation more recently are becoming interested in the colored population, and have come to realize their need of assistance," wrote May Mann Jennings, the president of the Florida Federation of Women's Clubs.[95]

Foote demonstrated from the start that the nursing program offered its services to African Americans. A Virginia doctor remarked that the only way for an African American to get treatment for tuberculosis was "to commit a felony, steal a horse, or break into a house before he had any chance to get well from consumption,"[96] yet Florida's open-air treatment was available to all. State health nurses treated African American patients, visited schools, and worked with African American clubwomen to establish antituberculosis societies. In the segregated South it was "unlawful to require any white female nurse to nurse in wards or rooms in hospitals, either public or private in which negro men are placed," and the law required every institution to employ "colored nurses to care for colored patients," but public health measures brought the races together.[97] Away from the confines of the institutions' physical constructions such as nursing schools or hospitals, the state health nurses could adopt a more inclusive path.

Florida's state health officials echoed Terry's reasoning to justify reaching out to the black population. African Americans, they argued, were the cause of disease. "The undue morbidity of the State of Florida is chargeable in large part to the ignorance and lack of right living on the part of the negro population," declared the public health evaluator Fox. "It is therefore obvious that the work of the health officer is required among the negroes as well as the whites . . . not only to prevent the spread of the disease to the white population, but also to conserve the life and health of the laboring classes of the South, upon whose physical fitness many industries depend." Fox recommended the appointment of "some colored nurses . . . who can carry on work among their own people to advantage," but the board appointed only one, Lottie Culp Gantt (b. 1887). While the board assigned each white state nurse a district, it employed Gantt to solely address the African American neighborhoods and "supplement the work of the white nurses among her own race."[98] The idea that black nurses were more suited to travel and attend to black patients in rural areas fed into one of the most abhorrent and damaging Jim Crow customs that spoke to the fears of biological mixing—that white nurses might be in danger from men of color.[99]

In the reports, Gantt's inclusion as the lone black nurse was readily identifiable. The white nurses were listed with their marital status, using the common title of "Miss" or "Mrs." As a black nurse, Gantt was afforded no title, in an overt Jim Crow–era slight.[100] The policy of referring to black graduate nurses as "Nurse" instead of "Miss" or "Mrs." was a code commonly adopted in white newspapers, the *American Journal of Nursing*, and other publications as well as in everyday practice. The code marginalized black nurses and bore consequences that affected their lives and career choices. The black press and the National Association of Colored Graduate Nurses made no such distinction between black and white nurses.

For the association, Gantt's employment was a double-edge sword. She had the distinction of becoming the first African American state nurse but was not a graduate of a nursing school. Born in Jacksonville, she was the daughter of the schoolteacher Mary Emily Jefferson Culp and Dr. Daniel W. Culp, a minister and physician, who served as superintendent of the Negro State League for the Prevention of Tuberculosis. Lottie Culp Gantt undertook most of her work in the African American neighborhoods of Tampa, where the poorest people lived in makeshift timber shacks with small yards, outdoor privies, and water pumps. She engaged the interest of clubwomen who in turn demonstrated an interest in her work by forming health committees to help, as Gantt put it, to "give more attention to the suffering."[101] During the 1916 white clubwomen's convention, May Mann Jennings led a discussion of health work and club work "among negroes, followed by . . . a report . . . [of] work among the colored clubs in Tampa."[102]

As a teacher, Gantt was particularly interested in the African American schools, which were ill equipped, overcrowded, and in great need of uplift; one-fourth of black children in Tampa between the ages of six and eighteen did not attend school. The legislature did not provide adequate resources to educate African American children; in fact, no one seemed to "care for the poor negro and his neglected school."[103] The lack of support for black schools was in part due to concern that educated African Americans would become more educated and wealthy than white citizens.[104] While the conditions of the black schools were deplorable, there was also much neglect in the white schools. The Florida Federation of Women's Clubs mobilized its members to take action to address schoolchildren's health and environment, and in 1915 a law was passed to provide for the health supervision of all schoolchildren. State nurses had also noted the need for sanitation in schools and the lack of medical inspectors to examine schoolchildren. Gantt believed the shortcomings opened the door for her future work as a health educator. "I note a great deficiency of sanitary methods and such little knowledge on the part of children as to the essentials of sound health," she wrote in her report to Porter offering to take on further responsibility to educate children on health matters. If humble in her request to Porter to perform the work—"I would like, if it is alright with you, ask that I may"—she foresaw that her instructions would yield results "effecting a general awakening among the children."[105] Gantt's expectation to perform such work for the state was unprecedented.

The board's reasoning to employ Gantt may have been in response to Fox's recommendation, but its willingness to provide health care to African Americans was not. While other southern states built segregated sanitariums, in Florida black and white nurses worked together and in collaboration with clubwomen to deliver a surprisingly inclusive service to rural communities.[106] In the black neighborhoods of Daytona and Ormond Beach, Irene Foote reported on the desperate need for a full-time, dedicated public health nurse.

Mary McLeod Bethune had long advocated for nurses to reach into the underserved districts. "There is a colored hospital in connection with the Mary Bethune Industrial School, where the girls from the school are being sent out to care for the poorer negroes in their homes," Foote reported, assessing that the work required reinforcement.[107] The work "was not efficient service or systematic," she pointed out. Foote arranged for clubwomen, the Mary Bethune Industrial School, the Daytona city council, and philanthropists to contribute funds to provide for an African American public health nurse to serve the area. Foote followed up with the newly appointed public health nurse, and they visited the African American communities together. She concluded, "I find much good had been accomplished by her systematic visits and instructions."[108]

In West Palm Beach, Foote addressed similar problems, most critically "the lack of care for colored tuberculosis patients," and again worked with clubwomen as well as the city council to provide outdoor accommodation for patients either in tents or outdoor sleeping porches. According to Foote, many more patients were learning to sleep with their windows open. The fresh air treatment required considerable skill to encourage patients to comply, especially when many had "never before heard of such a thing."[109] Other state nurses too appealed to doctors to report the whereabouts of those in need regardless of race. Jessie Wheeler found that "many of the physicians do not help as much as they could do, by getting names and addresses of cases of tuberculosis among the colored people. They say negroes come to see them maybe once or twice, and then they do not see them again, and that they don't feel like bothering with them in anyway. I feel they could help me locate more cases if they only would do so." Still other nurses like Mary Roach made a point of discussing their outreach to educate the black and white communities. Roach celebrated "'Tuberculosis Week' with talks to the public and school children, both white and colored." Working with Gantt in Tampa, Harriet Sherman supported plans to initiate a "Colored Tuberculosis Society."[110]

A Roadblock to Professionalization

There was a roadblock in Foote's and her colleagues' drive to professionalize nursing, and that lay in Porter's reluctance to solely employ graduate nurses as the state's first public health nurses. Foote and Paschall had taken leading roles in the professionalization of nursing in the state. Both were members of the State Board of Examiners of Nurses, which was tightening the registration for all nurses permitted to practice in the state. Although the State Board of Health hired several qualified nurses including Foote and Paschall, others were appointed on their experience as instructors, not their nursing training. Leaders of the State Graduate Nurses Association voiced disagreement, noting that the move undercut the nursing registration law and their efforts at professionalization more generally. The State Board of Health viewed the work in terms of public housekeeping, not professional expertise.

Porter countered the Graduate Nurses Association's objections by arguing that hiring nongraduate nurses had a precedent. He cited the membership requirements of the American Public Health Association, noting that many of the men employed by that organization did not hold medical degrees.[111] In fact, the National Organization for Public Health Nursing followed suit by extending membership to laypersons to ensure the involvement and loyalty of the private citizens who financially supported public health endeavors and nursing programs.[112] But Porter's analogy was not valid. Laypersons were indeed an important component of the "three-horse" public health team, but they were not substitutes for scientifically trained doctors or nurses. On one hand, the State Board of Health placed its new appointees at the forefront of the antituberculosis crusade. On the other, it failed to acknowledge professional, graduate nurses as trained experts delivering a public health service.

Leaders within the State Graduate Nurses Association based their objection on what Karen Buhler-Wilkinson has described as an increasing problem when public health nursing was growing outside the control of the nursing profession. As the demand for public health nursing increased and visiting nursing agencies multiplied, the administrations led by lay philanthropists sidestepped nursing oversight. Ignoring the need to include nursing superintendents in these organizations led to bypassing the need to set nursing standards.[113] Foote was the only one who had attended a postgraduate public health course, at Teachers College in New York. It was the foremost institution to provide guidelines and the promise to establish a vital connection between visiting nursing and public health.[114] Local training programs conducted by visiting nurses associations, health departments, and nursing organizations, however, offered little to prepare the increasing numbers of public health nurses of the North, West, and South for their new role in disease prevention and left most to learn on the job. Foote and her graduate nurse colleagues believed public health nursing combined therapeutic and educational goals on individual and group levels, but Porter did not agree.

Rather than the descriptor "nurse," Porter declared that the terms "district sociological worker" and "tuberculosis instructor" more aptly described the women's new roles as "tuberculosis specialists." He finally settled on the inclusive title "district nurses" even though five women were not graduate nurses, but confusion remained.[115] Porter's assistant clarified the board's decision, stating that "the term 'nurse' as applied to the district sociological and sanitary instructor is a misnomer, as actual nursing care is seldom rendered, the chief function of these public health nurses being educational."[116] To ensure that the new workers were all well versed in the tenets of preventive medicine and sufficiently prepared in their role as bridges, the board required Florida's first state health nurses to pass its own stringent examination.

The recruitment of nurses added the issue of class to another layer of insight into the State Board of Health's push to provide public health intercessions to the state. The board stated that the purpose of the examination was to select the "best informed in this line of work" from the large number of candidates. The three examiners appointed to determine the best informed did not include a nurse leader, a further point that undercut the burgeoning nursing profession. Dr. R. H. McGinnis of Jacksonville was "well known" to Porter and appointed the chairman. Dr. Ellen Lowell-Stevens was "most competent by reason of her professional education and connection with the Women's Clubs." Completing the trio was Marcus Fagg, "an enthusiastic social worker, in charge of the Children's Home Society."[117]

While all the nurses passed the requisite written examination and their selection was based on their experience as instructors, not their nursing training, there was also an unreported quality. As the prerequisite for the new roles was not a nursing qualification, the board noted that "favoritism, friendship or political preferment [would] not be permitted to influence the selection." Contrary to the board's statement, the recruitment reflected that the selection of non-nurses was, indeed, women who were well known to members of the board and with social standing in their communities.[118] Frances Herndone was the board's librarian, and Laura Scott was a leader in the Women's Christian Temperance Union. Elsie Forrest and the lone African American, Lottie Culp Gantt, were teachers and daughters of prominent physicians, Dr. J. D. Forrest of Bradentown and Dr. Daniel W. Culp of Jacksonville. Jessie Wheeler, the nurse who did not graduate from a nursing school, joined her sister, Lydia Kirk, who was among the first cohort of nurses to graduate in 1895 from the first class of Florida's first nursing school, at St. Luke's Hospital in Jackson-

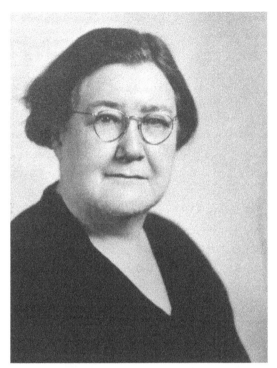

Figure 1.3. Jessie Wheeler joined her sister, Lydia Kirk, as one of the first state health nurses, ca. 1916. Courtesy of Gail VanderVoort.

ville. She was married to the pharmacist James Edgar Kirk. Of the nurses, a newcomer from Illinois, Susan Voorhees, was the wife of Warder Voorhees, the board's first statistician. Foote, of course, had already made a name for herself with Jacksonville's City Board of Health and the State Graduate Nurses Association of Florida. Like many others in the North, she was one who saw the problem of excluding nursing leadership from the development of public health nursing.[119] But as the history unfolded, the short term of the district nurses' employment thwarted her attempts to influence Florida's State Board of Health in significant ways.

Much of the board's confusion about the new field of public health nursing was, perhaps, more in line with the traditional conception of nurses as deferential helpmeets or as one doctor put it, the physician's "chief assistant" and "truest friend."[120] The public health nurses represented something quite different; they were progressive, autonomous professionals who made decisions about public health and rural patients independently. Some local physicians were impressed by the likes of Foote and her colleagues and worked collaboratively on public health initiatives, while others held tight to their conservative beliefs and their medical records. Susan Voorhees was able to win over the physicians in her district: "I am no longer treated with indifference, and the work referred to as a joke, but with respect, and as a co-worker, an ally, and not a meddlesome rival." Irene Foote turned two "antagonistic" doctors into "staunch supporters of the movement," but Laura Scott branded her district's physicians as "extremely indifferent and unconcerned." Mary Spencer, who had joined forces with local women's clubs to secure reports on tubercular patients, was not surprised that the doctors did not comply. Even the weight of the clubwomen's presence did little to encourage these country doctors to collaborate with the board's initiatives. "We had not one response," Spencer reported. "The women were discouraged, but I was not surprised. The doctors seem unwilling to report cases to a nurse."[121] Porter was not surprised either. "I am inclined to believe that very little active co-operation may be expected from the physicians as a whole," he conceded.[122]

By late 1916 the populist candidate Sidney J. Catts (1863–1936) was unbeatable in the race for governor, and Porter expected the board's budget to come under scrutiny.[123] In November the state nurses' automobile privileges were revoked, leaving them stranded at headquarters. Sherman was clear. There was no way to reach rural patients without an automobile. She forcefully recommended "allowance made if only a limited amount, for automobile hire as there are patients in secluded districts who have no physicians, and it is impossible to get a horse, even if it is obtainable." And to give her request further weight she added, "It is not safe for a woman to go alone to drive such a distance."[124] Yet the state nurses did travel great distances, often alone and often at the wheel of automobiles that provided a "new, movable field" to facilitate getting their work done.[125] "Automobiles for the individual workers will be the only way we can carry on the visits in a satisfactory way to any of the rural cases or country schools," wrote a frustrated Foote. "As it is now, we will only be able to reach the larger communities and visit the few patients living in town."[126] Foote's future plans were also in jeopardy.

Purportedly the state could not find the budget to continue the promising state health nursing program.[127] Defunding the positions of all the nurses gutted the momentum of the board's incentives to reach the rural population. "It is a great blow to our work," complained Dr. Grace Whitford, expressing her dismay on behalf of the clubwomen. It is "a great setback, [because] the Federation has worked a great many years for the establishment and increase of this service."[128] Porter "was not in sympathy" with the new administration and handed in his resignation on March 23, 1917.[129] In concert with the United States' entry into World War I, Porter and many of Florida's state health nurses traded in their public health work for wartime service.[130]

Speaking from her clubwoman's platform, Whitford appealed for graduate nurses to take up the field of public health nursing and continue the progressive precedent to provide a service for the rural and African American poor. "This type of woman is, perhaps, our greatest need throughout the state, in every county," she concluded.[131] State leadership in public health nursing did not return to Florida until 1922, when Laurie Jean Reid became the director of Florida's Bureau of Child Welfare. In the interim, counties including Hillsborough, Dade, and Pinellas answered Whitford's call—and Foote's—to appoint public health nurses. Some were employed through a Red Cross funding campaign in collaboration with the clubwomen, others by the recently formed Florida Anti-Tuberculosis Association. And still others were hired by parent-teacher associations that funded school nurses in several districts.[132] After the war, greater inroads to serve the rural areas and the African American communities sprouted from northern leadership through the Red Cross and the National Health Circle for Colored People. These organizations would eventually run parallel to the new state health nursing program and begin to answer Rosa Williams Brown's call that black graduate nurses be tasked with the obligation to care for the health of the black population.

From her base at the Provident Hospital in Jacksonville, Brown observed the inclusion of Gantt as a state health nurse and the obstacles white nurses encountered on their road to professional development. As an outsider within the graduate nursing body in Florida, she also observed the source of power and authority that white nurses believed they had mustered. Yet she witnessed Foote's failure to organize a public health nursing association for Florida as well as the State Graduate Nurses Association's inability to reverse Porter's decision to employ nongraduate nurses. Successful or not, white nurses had a voice to object to the board's action. The black nurses' lack of voice spurred Brown to action.[133] In 1916 she took measures to organize a local association for black graduate nurses, believing it was a step forward in their professionalization, "for in union there is strength," she wrote.[134] But there were still too few homegrown black graduates eligible to join Brown's local effort. It was left up to her and another diehard strong leader, Petra Pinn, a 1906 graduate from Tuskegee, who became the first superintendent of the recently opened Pine Ridge Hospital in West Palm Beach to strengthen Florida's ties with the National Association of Colored Graduate Nurses. They surveyed the need to strengthen nursing schools, and they pressed graduates to "wake up to the importance of registration." Quietly and firmly, like many of their counterparts in the South, they negotiated how best to bridge their work and deliver much-needed health intercessions to the rural and poor urban communities of Florida.

2

||||||||||||||||||||||||||||||||||||||||||||||||||||||||||||||||||||||||

Stirring Northern Initiatives into
Florida's Backwaters, 1922 to 1930

||||||||||||||||||||||||||||||||||||||||||||||||||||||||||||||||||||||||

On March 7, 1923, six months after she arrived in Florida to become the director of the State Board of Health's Bureau of Child Welfare and public health
nursing, Laurie Jean Reid took up her pen to sketch her perspective on the
intertwining problems of race and poverty that mired Florida in its backward-
ness. Her confidential letter to Grace Abbot, chief of the federal Children's
Bureau, was a "word picture" of her job and an outline of the future work
necessary if she was to lead the board's public health nurses to save lives. "So
much of Florida is rural and not easy of access by road or railroad, and the
distribution of physicians in the State is confined principally to the large towns
and settlements," she wrote, making it clear that the public health nurses were
of the utmost importance to seeking out those sidelined by doctors. "A great
proportion of the obstetrical work is done by midwives who are the same type
that I found in such numbers in Mississippi when I began to work there,"
continued Reid, reminding Abbott about her previous assignment for the
Children's Bureau when she conducted a survey of midwives in Mississippi.[1]
Florida, Mississippi, and the rest of the South required solutions for the high
infant and maternal mortality that contrasted dismally with those of many
European countries.[2] Florida was home to "the same type of midwives, who
performed the majority of the deliveries," Reid wrote. With a tone of professional arrogance she added, "My nurses have found up to the present time over
two thousand, none of whom have what you or I would call training for their
work and the majority are illiterate, ignorant negro women." Reid poured out

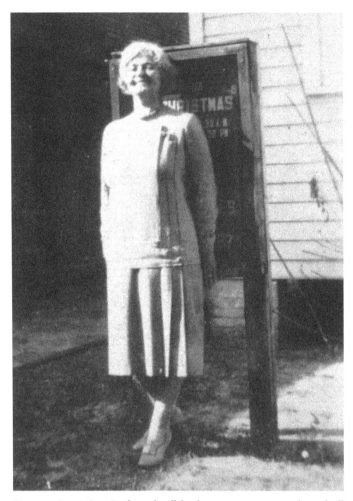

Figure 2.1. Laurie Jean Reid stands tall for the camera, ca. 1929, and stood tall during her tenure in Florida as the state's director of public health nursing from 1922 to 1929. Courtesy of the American College of Nurse Midwives and the National Library of Medicine.

her impatience with the deficiency of health reform in the state and her lack of sympathy for mothers and midwives who were grounded in poverty and lacked medical care and knowledge to preserve the health of their families and clients. She confided, "Personally, I loathe the midwife, and would be glad if we can have what I am firmly convinced every woman ought to have, a trained obstetrician, under whose care she should be from the moment she knows she is pregnant until she is safely over the first month following the delivery." Reid asserted to Abbott that such a standard was impossible to set "when it will be years and years before anything of the sort can even be thought of for our State."[3] Reid's words set the stage to examine why it would be years and years before anything of that sort could be thought of for African American women. In fact, Reid's assumptions point to the cultural construction of health in the midwifery program as she began to lay the groundwork for the consequences it entailed.

Reed's tenure in Florida began on September 15, 1922, after Governor Cary A. Hardee accepted the terms of the Sheppard-Towner Maternity and Infancy Protection Act prior to its ratification by the state legislature.[4] Congress passed the Sheppard-Towner Act in 1921,[5] two years after the Nineteenth Amendment enfranchised women in an achievement that directly reflected the new political power of women and the propulsion of issues of special import to women.[6] The purpose of the act was to fund states' projects to promote the health and welfare of mothers and infants. States with different maternal and child health issues would decide how best to arrange for cooperation between public health authorities, physicians, nurses, and other reformers. Most generally the goals were to promote birth registration, establish infant welfare and maternity centers, and provide classes for midwives and mothers.[7] Florida was one of the fourteen states with the highest maternal and infant mortality rates, confirming the necessity to include "licensing, inspecting, supervising and instructing of midwives."[8] The act provided for federal matching funds to states that designated a state agency to provide maternity and preschool programs with nutrition and hygiene instruction and prenatal and child health clinics.[9] Reid, as the director of the state agency, delivered monthly reports and accounting to the Children's Bureau Board of Maternal and Infant Hygiene of the US Department of Labor, which was responsible for the administration and implementation of the act. She was fired up with a reformer's vision to provide expert administration of the program, but she recognized that bringing federal initiatives into a state would be an uphill climb.[10] "If we expect to get anything, and take care of women in the meantime," Reid wrote to Abbott, "I constantly uphold the ideal [of health reform] towards which we must work both to my nurses, the lay people in the communities, the midwives and everyone [with] whom we come in contact in a professional way but while we are upholding this ideal, we must begin with 'what we've got, where we're at.'"[11]

As a newcomer to the state, Reid soon discovered that "what she got" was valuable support from the women's clubs to sway the legislature to accept the Sheppard-Towner Act.[12] Although Governor Hardee unofficially accepted the terms of the act, official acceptance was dependent on the endorsement from Florida's legislature during the 1923 session. This was a requirement for eligibility to receive the appropriation of federal funds, but as the legislature was not responsive to the state's public health initiatives, one of Reid's first tasks was to campaign for its acceptance and call on clubwomen to "exert their influence towards having the legislature accept the federal aid."[13] Florida clubwomen's support for the Sheppard-Towner Act was in concert with their previous work to develop the field of public health nursing and to demand that the Florida legislature address the health and welfare of the state's children. Their concern for Florida's children contributed to the establishment of the State Board of Health's Bureau of Child Welfare in 1918.[14] However, since there were no state health nurses to implement the bureau's policy and with almost no financial backing from the state, the bureau's ineffectiveness only strengthened the clubwomen's resolve to support the Sheppard-Towner Act. Florida's clubwomen were among the flood of reforming women to endorse the bill in 1918 when it was introduced into the House of Representatives by Jeanette Rankin, the first congresswoman.[15] They remained stalwart supporters and backed Reid to ensure that the Florida legislature accept the terms of the Sheppard-Towner Act.[16] Still, Reid faced tough opposition. State Senators John P. Stokes, William C. Hodges, and John B. Johnson revisited the arguments submitted in the congressional debate earlier by declaring that the approval to accept federal funds would be "another surrender of States rights."[17]

Such opposition to the acceptance of the act brought out Reid's fire. She dismissed those who argued against the intrusion of the federal government into state affairs, claiming opponents were ignorant of the poor standards of health and the "toll of infant deaths and maiming due to unnecessary blindness."[18] From one enthusiastic speech to another, Reid rallied the clubwomen with passion, gesticulating and becoming dramatic as she delineated the necessity for midwife education. Prominent clubwomen like May Mann Jennings answered her call. Collaboration with Jennings was especially important, as she had spearheaded a new force, the Florida Legislative Council, a "clearing house" to accommodate all issues of legislative importance to women's associations and clubs. The Florida Legislative Council acted in concert with the Florida League of Women Voters to support Reid's efforts and persuade the legislature to accept the requirements of the act.[19] Their work came to fruition on May 7, 1923, when the legislature accepted the terms and it became state law. Reform-minded women had done their part. Next Reid turned her attention to its implementation, which rested in large measure with her team of public health nurses and educating the public on the work they would accomplish.

"A public health nurse is both a nurse and a teacher," wrote Reid in *Florida Health Notes*, aiming to educate Florida's public about the new profession for women that had gathered impetus after World War I. It had become "an indispensable instrument in every modern health movement," she pointed out, implying that Florida lagged behind the national momentum. She was positioned to implement the new program for Florida and from the onset expected readers to pick up that her efficient management would strengthen the profession of public health nursing for the whole state and begin to transform the local situation. "We should make provision for those to do the permanent work who are well qualified by personality, education and training," she wrote. If her goal was to promote the public health nurse of Florida to become a "recognized factor in community welfare," her immediate task was to sell the concept to community leaders.

Reid adopted gendered language to stress that the nature of the public health nurses' work did not deviate from a female nurse's traditional qualities. A public health nurse is first "a woman with a woman's heart big enough to take in every suffering, helpless bit of humanity and give it skilled care," she wrote, expecting that such terms would make the nurses' new roles acceptable to the community.[20] Her statement fed into prevailing conservative mindsets like that of the Floridian Dr. John Boyd, a surgeon who spoke at the first annual convention of the State Graduate Nurses Association of Florida a decade earlier: "The nurse ought to be *a woman*, first, last and always . . . the sexes both have their sphere in this life . . . A nurse is not a nurse until she is first a woman—first, last and always, so, I say, be a woman."[21] To be sure, Boyd's words mirrored others throughout the nation betraying an anxiety about the new paths women sought in public life. Reid understood the rhetoric of control and sought to reassure the public that even though these new roles were backed with professional training and education they were indeed womanly. And in their prescriptive roles they would proceed to chart their courses even as doing so required "courage" and a "pioneer spirit."[22] Reid's intent to note the pioneer spirit was yet another suggestion that Florida was behind its northern contemporaries. Reid's tone served her purpose to promote the new profession—and herself. She had epitomized how her professional training, pioneering spirit, and determination to blaze a trail in Florida brought her to the state in the first place.

Born Laurie Jean Sheperd on October 3, 1884, in Ontario, Canada, Reid changed her name upon marriage sometime before 1906 when she graduated from the Clara Barton Memorial School for Nurses in Los Angeles. Naturalized in 1911, she began to advance her career in public health during World War I when she was either widowed or divorced. Under the auspices of the Red Cross Nursing Service, she made a name for herself in leadership positions first in Alabama and then in Georgia, so when the US Public Health Service organized the third federal nursing service in 1919, Reid became the chief nurse at the Office of Industrial Hygiene in Washington, DC.[23] In 1920 the Public Health Service sent her west, to Montana's State Board of Health to become the director of child welfare. There she learned that bringing about change was dependent upon arousing the public's interest in her work and gaining the support of clubwomen. Reid's next assignment, in Mississippi, brought her in contact with midwives. After an extensive survey, Reid declared that the high infant and maternal mortality rates in Mississippi were due to negligent physicians as well as illiterate and ignorant midwives. Similar to Terry's stance toward midwives in Jacksonville, Reid disregarded the issue of substandard physician care because public health officials believed it would be counterproductive to criticize physicians.[24] She believed the midwives were an easier target to address in Mississippi, as they would be in Florida. Experience gained in Mississippi, Montana, Alabama, and Georgia provided the grounding to drive Reid's strategies in Florida. Her immediate goal was to establish authority over the midwives and bring health enlightenment to the mothers they served. Her training and prior experience in public health was laced with a large dose of cultural chauvinism, an ingredient that pitted white professionals against the superstitious black midwives and poor rural women both black and white.[25]

Reid required a strong team of state health nurses who understood Florida's culture and environment and the work they faced in the neglected rural and urban areas. She noted that the supervision of midwives was only undertaken by the health departments of the larger cities "if the health officers were sufficiently interested."[26] The initial field staff consisted of four graduate nurses with public health experience, three white and one black, who were well grounded in the local situation. Harriet J. Sherman was the most experienced in Florida's public health practices. She was one of the first three state health nurses to work for the State Board of Health in 1914 and excelled at spelling out the depth of her experience when speaking to clubwomen and informing them about the benefits of the Sheppard-Towner Act. "Miss Sherman's hearers felt that her words were authority because of her experiences in this work, she having handled over 3,500 babies in clinics and otherwise," the *Tampa Tribune* reported. "She is now conducting a clinic in Brooksville and scores of Hernando county babies have been examined."[27] The three remaining nurses were also strong candidates to work in the state's unique environment. Prior to her arrival in Florida, Noreita M. Alvis (1889–1957) was the supervisor of public health nursing in Richmond, Virginia, when Ruth Mettinger joined her staff. Born in Florida in 1896, Mettinger went north to Roxborough School of Nursing in Pennsylvania and on to Erie for her first public health experience. Under Alvis, her work in Virginia with midwives followed and prepared her for her appointment in Florida.

The only African American on the staff was Estelle Evans Bonner (b. 1894) born in Florida and a 1914 graduate of Jacksonville's Brewster Hospital School of Nursing. Just as race separated Lottie Culp Gantt, the board's lone black nurse in 1916, race also separated the Sheppard-Towner Act nurses. Reid assigned Bonner to work in sixteen counties of northwest and north central Florida, a region known as Florida's Black Belt. And again, the board's commitment to assign a black nurse to address the black community spoke to the larger issues of scientific racism and the fear of biological mixing. Reid did not single out specific instructions to Bonner but noted more generally that as the state was "largely rural," demonstrations made in one community would have little influence in another. With Bonner covering the poorest counties of the state, the Sheppard-Towner team began their fieldwork for the whole state with an understanding of Florida's country life, country folk, and racial ideology—an understanding, Reid noted, that would not be grasped by nurses from the North.[28]

The Challenges of the Local Situation

In her letter to Abbott, Reid bluntly laid out the reasons the Sheppard-Towner Act nurses' work in Florida was so difficult. It was not simply geography or landscape, but the social and biological fears created by Jim Crow customs. Between the lines of her letter, she revealed her anxiety as she set the scene of working in the presence of racial tension. Amplifying the difficulty of introducing new ideas to a people set in their long-established way of life, she referenced lynching. "We would not dare mention Prenatal Clinics or we'd run the risk of being lynched," she wrote.[29] In Florida between 1918 and 1927, there were forty-seven people lynched and numerous incidents of mob violence during which houses were torched and property was destroyed.[30] There can be little doubt that many African Americans fled the state after World War I not just for economic reasons but also to escape the real or imagined mounting violence threatened by the violent white mobs and the Ku Klux Klan. Tensions between the races exploded throughout the South, fired up, in part, by accounts in local white newspapers that promulgated the alleged racial attacks on white women and the fear of black men carrying weapons to protect themselves. Reid's work began in the wake of one of the well-publicized accounts in southern and northern newspapers about the mob-induced Rosewood massacre in rural Levy County following an alleged rape of a white woman by a black man. The violence that followed resulted in at least eight deaths, the black township of Rosewood burned down, and its residents driven out forever. The violence was a striking example of racial tension that had boiled over and could not be ignored by the state health nurses in the field.[31] The background of such violence influenced Reid's language. Although in the records there appear to be no references to any lynching or mob violence directly observed by any state health nurse, the presence of it surely cast a pall on their work.

Reid's graphic image highlighted the difficulty of reaching women to counsel about prenatal care, but her job was to seek solutions. She explained to Abbott how she circumvented the threat by masking the introduction of prenatal care. She arranged for baby clinics where local physicians performed infant examinations assisted by the state health nurses. The nurses then had a route to do follow-up work seeking the mothers in their homes and in more intimate settings learn which mothers might be expecting babies. The dual purpose of the baby clinics was a starting point, a means to get to know the mothers, but as Reid outlined, it was "the longest way round for the shortest way home." Reid seemed to reassure herself as well as inform Abbott that with continual effort, she could bring change to mothers. She wrote, "If we can keep our vision and maintain strength sufficient to keep eternally at it, we will eventually get there."[32]

The goal of saving mothers' and infants' lives opened the opportunity for Reid to criticize the local situation and express her exasperation at the way of life for rural women. In one passionate speech to clubwomen she "flayed" rural motherhood in her attempt to highlight the childbirth and child-rearing practices among country people. She complained that poor Floridian mothers saw their continual round of childbirth at a young age as perfectly natural, and she spoke graphically against such practices: "The first thing you know you have a dead mother and baby or else the two in such poor health they might just as well be dead."[33] Her firsthand observations of the profound ills that perpetuated women's cycle of poverty fell in line with other contemporary critics. The sociologist Margaret Jarman Hagood has concluded that it was the "culturally inherited ideology that [held] mothers to their tasks and in their places with the sanction of God and the Southern tradition." For these mothers, "intellectual contemplation" was not possible. There was no education, no time, and no financial relief. Moreover, rural isolation prevented contact with other people.[34] Daughters "brought up right" followed the pattern set in their childhood. Early marriage, sometimes as young as thirteen years, repeated the cycle of the culture—and poverty.[35]

Reid's judgment on the poor outlook for such mothers and babies reflected the eugenic philosophy that had found favor in the Progressive Era with many public health advocates including the nurse leader Lavinia Dock.[36] Proponents advocated "the development of the human race under favorable physical, economic and social conditions."[37] Reid disseminated her views to readers of *Florida Health Notes*: "Infant mortality is the most sensitive index we possess of social welfare. . . . [I]t measures the intelligence, health, and right living of fathers and mothers and the standards of morals and sanitation of communities and governments." She backed up her points in the article by quoting the eminent pediatrician Emmett Holt's words: "Does God fix the death rate? . . . We are now beginning to look upon infant mortality as evidence of human weakness, ignorance and stupidity."[38] In her flaying of motherhood, Reid poured out her frustration with country women and the difficulties of introducing new ideas to a people wedded to tradition and set in their ways. At the same time, she once again underscored her professional prejudice.

For Reid the cultural aspects of the local situation marked Florida as a backward state. The practice of midwifery performed outside the boundaries of professional medicine was absolutely against the ideals of her training as a public health nurse.[39] Like many of her counterparts striving for midwifery reform in the South, Reid concluded that midwives were a necessary evil.[40] As she considered the midwives not only illiterate but also ignorant, she devised a plan of education. "It is one thing to lay down laws and say that a certain standard must be maintained in various kinds of work, but it seems foolish to me to try to maintain a standard which goes over the heads of the people with whom one must work," she insisted."[41] She began by writing a pictorial manual to guide midwives, noting to Abbott that educational literature provided by the Children's Bureau "did not fit the local situation."[42] Since Florida's law to license midwives did not come to fruition until 1931, Reid arranged for the board to issue "certificates of fitness" to the trustworthy midwives. Such innovations were made necessary by the failure of the legislature to support midwifery reform.[43] While the nature of Reid's work in relation to the population she served demanded professional authority, the success in reducing infant and maternal mortality rates depended upon her ability to translate the goals of medical reform to underprivileged women and lay midwives. Lasting accomplishments were best reached by involving the women and midwives themselves to become active participants to address maternal and infant mortality.[44] Yet as the objective success of the program depended upon how she directed that perspective in her everyday work, her language of continually dehumanizing the midwife mattered. Her nurses, she wrote, were busily engaged in "rounding up what midwives they could reach."[45]

Compounding the cultural problems of the local situation were the physical difficulties to reach the midwives, mothers, and children amid weather-related concerns, bad roads, and poor access to out-of-the-way places. The majority of midwives lived in country places that were least accessible. Mothers, too, were hard to reach, whether they worked in the strawberry fields or attended the "epidemic of revivals" that kept them busy sometimes with three meetings a day. "Torrential rains," "roads impassable," and "travel hard" appeared frequently in Reid's reports. The Florida Keys were difficult to visit with only one train in twenty-four hours and only one stop, at Knight's Key, prior to reaching Key West. At Port Washington and Santa Rosa in Walton County, nurses hired boats to reach the "out of the way places." In the Everglades community at Moore Haven, conditions were so bad the land was flooded for three successive years. Reid was forced to come to terms with her ideal of efficiency to justify the time necessary to travel to the sparsely populated places. She acknowledged that some might question whether the nurses' time was well spent to reach the remote locations. Spending a whole day to visit just a few children was not a "waste of time," she insisted. The value of the work, Reid concluded, was not a measurable statistic. It could not be measured by the volume "but by the good done."[46] At every opportunity Reid championed the cause that had quickly become hers. The state health nurses "drove along bad roads, walked across prairie and boggy paths, coped with rain and missed ferry connections but when they finally reached their destination, they were bound to succeed since [they] refuse . . . to recognize obstacles," she wrote in 1926 for *Florida Health Notes*—almost echoing Porter's assessment of the first state health nurses' work in 1914.[47] Meeting the challenges of the local situation then became not only a test of Reid's judgment but also a trial of how well the Sheppard-Towner nurses effectively imposed rules and regulations to a mostly rural population without creating racial and class tension.

Meeting the Challenges with an "Elastic Plan"

Reid implemented what she called a "very elastic plan" to try out various experiments of work and find the best fit for the local situation. Each Sheppard-Towner nurse spent approximately one week in each county, with Bonner covering the Black Belt. In advance of their visits, the state health nurses sent letters to local physicians, any public health nurses who might already be employed in the area, and any interested persons to explain the purpose of the Maternal and Infant Hygiene program. Ideally, the state health nurses arrived in an area with a certain amount of fanfare to promote the program and reach a broader community. The first hurdle to overcome was to adjust the clinic days to best suit the rural people. Saturday was "the best day for colored people since that was the day they always come into towns for their supplies . . . so whenever possible we use . . . Friday for white and Saturday for colored."[48] Publicity to advertise the clinics was necessary to reach the mothers and midwives and at the same time promote the work of the field staff.

Overcoming hurdles with midwife education was one of the main thrusts of the elastic plan. As it was often difficult to assemble the midwives together for classes, Reid reported more success in seeking out the midwives to give instruction and examination "in the midwife's home, or under a tree in the field, or where the midwife can be found. If we waited until all the midwives from any given section could be gotten together in class, we would never get work done."[49] Acknowledgment that midwives were "doing their best" to comply with instructions indicated a favorable response from the midwives and recognition of their efforts to raise their standards once provided with the necessary information. Reid's pictorial manual guided midwives to earn their certificates of fitness. According to Reid, those midwives who could not keep pace with the reformed methods were induced to cease their practice when advised to do so by the nurse, and they did so willingly. But this was an optimistic conclusion. Later accounts offered by the state health nurses call Reid's conclusion into question.[50]

The trial-and-error elastic plan proved a concrete effort to reach mothers as well as the midwives. Mothers did not passively accept middle-class ideals on childbearing and child rearing. Unlike midwives, who did not have a choice to accept or refuse their education, mothers were free to accept or refuse this governmental intrusion. Many were grateful for the health care but did not relinquish their traditional practices and beliefs.[51] Reid acknowledged that the nurses would have to find a means to gain the women's confidence to make changes. It was, she stated, "a difficult matter for a strange person, even though she be a woman and a professional one, to approach a prospective mother on so intimate a subject" as childbirth.[52]

Based on the state health nurses' outreach to mothers, Reid came to terms with how best to reach them, reporting that mothers were far more responsive to "neighborhood institutes," a type of informal gathering held separately for both African American and white mothers; these were more sociable than the formal instruction offered by the nurses in mothers' classes. The state health nurses learned that the most effective way to make maternal and infant demonstrations was to seek out a woman who was willing to offer her home for the meeting and to draw the crowd: "The woman herself invites friends and neighbors being left in control of the matter of whom might attend." The nurse could then begin her talk by telling women that "she wished to help them to learn to improvise in order to save money" and subsequently ease her way to instruct mothers in prenatal, postnatal, and child care. Previously the nurses had discovered that the mothers' sheer poverty had left them discouraged when they were overwhelmed by the "very excellence" of the nurses' demonstration equipment. Before the suggestion was made of expending a single penny, the nurses found that a far more effective way to get through to the mothers was to demonstrate how to use materials of things at hand, even the contents of a rag bag, in their preparation for childbirth.[53] This informal technique proved beneficial. In this instance the nurses recognized the promotion of middle-class conveniences, not values, were at issue and beyond the reach of most women.

Obstacles surfaced in birth registration when the state nurses found that physicians were more reluctant to comply with the instructions than the midwives were. "Physicians seem to be the ones who are hardest to make reports of their births," Reid complained. Even though some physicians were grateful for the support of the state health nurses to assist them with their records, others were "antagonistic to the work." Once again Reid relied on collaboration with clubwomen to help the nurses. She took credit for "inducing" the clubwomen to help, an attitude that seems to ignore their enthusiastic prior outreach. The intensive campaign over the summer, with the clubwomen "to add to its weight," yielded positive results. By September 1924 Reid reported that both physicians and midwives were more prompt in reporting births. On October 8, 1924, Florida was admitted to the Federal Birth Registration Area, after Mississippi (1921), South Carolina (1919), and Virginia (1917) but ahead of Alabama (1927), Tennessee (1927), and Georgia (1928).[54]

While orchestrating midwife and physician compliance toward birth registration, Reid continued to oversee routine work where state health nurses often worked without the assistance of physicians. In 1926, for example, an increased staff of state health nurses assisted doctors to conduct five child health conferences and inspect 476 children. On their own, however, the state health nurses conducted 254 child health conferences with "no physician present" and inspected 3,885 children.[55] There was no indication that Reid was explicitly critical of the physicians' neglect of public health, a pattern that was not unique to Florida. Nurses most often overlooked physicians' indifference and even hostility in the name of professional loyalty.[56] Rather than criticize the doctors, Reid saw the statistics as an indication of the strength of her bureau. "The most outstanding achievement of the year is the control of midwifery, educational and supervisory work in tourist camps, [and] education of the general public to the needs of mothers and children," she concluded.[57]

By the mid-1920s medical service to tourist camps marked Florida's distinctive position among the southern states. Many newcomers to the state were drawn by the prospects of a new life and new homes in what a headline in the *New York Times* touted as a "tropical empire."[58] Congested cities were unable to absorb the scores of visitors. Before the rise of motels, what were called "tin can tourist camps" sprouted up on the outskirts of Gainesville, Tampa, and Miami. Many more grew up in remote locations and off the beaten path. Reid described the congestion in one of her word pictures to Grace Abbott in 1925 that captured the momentum. "Every road coming into the state looks like a circus parade," she wrote, "or I think maybe a comparison of everyone going to a fire might be more exact. Every broken down Ford and wagon spilling over with children." It was obvious to Reid that the maternal and infant health program had to expand to serve the newcomers and visitors who arrived in the state with little more than their automobiles for shelter. "I realize that the work will be, maybe a disjointed, haphazard piece of work to outsiders but Florida certainly occupies a unique position among the states at present time," she concluded to Abbott.[59]

Reid voiced her concern that the transient nature of the camps would spike harmful consequences to their temporary residents and nearby communities. "Epidemics were bound to follow in the wake of these road travelers who accept no responsibility either for the community in which they pass a few days, the one they have left or to the one to which they are going," she reported. Reid illustrated her point with a description of her visit to one camp that offered graphic insight into the experiences of one young child who was "desperately ill in bed in a tent" before she could intervene to save the child's life. The tone in Reid's report to Abbott reflected her top-down attitude and impatience with what she perceived to be the mother's nonchalant attitude. "Close questioning of the mother brought no apparent reason for the raging fever or the intense pain in the head. The child did not want to be disturbed or touched, symptoms of grave significance to a professional person," she wrote. "The mother has made no effort to find a physician or get help of any kind although each case of illness in the camp is supposed to be reported to the camp manager at once." In Reid's assessment the situation was made even worse by "other children in this family who were out in the camp playing with children of other families." While holding the mother responsible, evidently Reid failed to see the situation from the mother's perspective. Just like the women who journeyed west on the overland trails seven decades earlier, these women travelers too left family, church, and community behind to embark on new lives in Florida. Undoubtedly this mother felt alone and isolated and had no one to turn to before Reid arrived. Reid's aim was clear. Her job was to save lives and prevent illness. Reid concluded that such cases must be "reported and properly cared for, but the possibility of other such cases not promptly or properly handled are the menace for which we must be constantly alert."[60]

Reid assigned two state health nurses to seek out the "floating populations" and provide prophylactic care before curative work became a necessity.[61] She was particularly anxious to reach out to mothers with babies and young children, pointing out that a consequence of the "tin can" diets left children malnourished. Before they could offer advice about nutrition and health, however, the nurses first had to convey compassion to overcome the mothers' suspicion and reticence.[62] From recommending the use of dried milk for the infants to teaching how best to avoid and/or rid families of hookworm and to maintaining vigilance for unhygienic conditions, the nurses' workload fit under the umbrella of the Sheppard-Towner Act's terms.[63] Avoiding disease and epidemics was an important health factor for everyone, but to accommodate for appropriation under the Sheppard-Towner terms, Reid related her goal to the Children's Bureau. Reporting her intent to Abbott Reid reiterated that her goal was "to save much of the suffering and possible death among mothers and little children by being on the job in the pioneer sections and this we propose to do and hope that you will approve."[64]

Expansion of Health Work

The success of the elastic plan helped Reid to portray herself as a confident leader willing to work around problems to implement change and to emphasize that the nurses under her direction were deterred by neither the environmental nor the social barriers the state imposed. Her leadership to build up the board's public health nursing department and provide leadership for public health nurses employed throughout the state had begun to reap results. In 1924 there were six Sheppard-Towner nurses and nine additional state health nurses to expand the field.[65] Reid made a point to clarify that the nurses paid for with Sheppard-Towner Act funds were employed only for infant and maternal work. In 1925 she began to see the results from her endeavors; she reported nineteen public health nurses under the Bureau of Child Welfare and additional new public health nursing services in eight counties and one city, Key West.[66] The following year Reid captured this new outreach and growing strength of public health nursing with a formal name change, to the Bureau of Child Hygiene and Public Health Nursing.[67]

Public health nurses employed by cities, counties, and various private concerns in the state looked to the bureau and Reid's leadership for guidance in their professional nursing practice. Up and down the state, from Defuniak Springs in Walton County to Vero Beach and on to Key West, Reid's and the state health nurses' continual petitions to counties, towns, and companies to employ public health nurses were backed by the Florida Federation of Women's Clubs and reaped results. Dr. M. Josie Rogers, the chair of the federation's Department of Public Welfare reiterated that public health nurses were often the only ones available to reach out with health interventions. She reported, "In many counties such a nurse is the only point of contact along health lines in child welfare work."[68] Reid was the liaison between the entities requiring the services of public health nurses and the nurses themselves. In Quincy, Gadsden County, she met with physicians and other local leaders to discuss public health issues and engage a county nurse.[69] In Pierce, Polk County, the American Agricultural Chemical Company secured an industrial nurse.[70] In Walton County, local communities hired their own public health nurse after Noreita Alvis promoted and exemplified "her excellent work" to begin the infant and maternity work in west Florida.[71] The national public health nurse leader Mary Gardner argued that waking up local leaders to the benefits a public health nurse could bring to the community would be a slow process, often taking "years and years of steady pressure . . . to produce results."[72] Reid was not willing to wait years and years. Her actions to encourage and promote the development of health programs in Florida showed her impatience to bring results.

Now with a larger staff of state health nurses, Reid continued her exhaustive attempts to promote public health measures throughout Florida. She was well positioned to forward a broad array of general programs and activities that required the nurses to drive the message home to the black and white communities. From rural Columbia and Suwannee Counties to the country areas near Orlando, rural people gathered at their respective segregated local schools for visits from the movie truck. Films on the importance of birth registration, mosquito control, child health, and the value of a public health nurse gave the state health nurses an opportunity for impromptu conferences.[73] May Day celebrations brought further opportunities to engage communities. Reid envisioned every community in the state, from "Pensacola to Key West," would take part in the celebrations; she declared, "The first of May is every child's day." To snap communities out of indifference, she encouraged their participation to help plan events and work toward her goal for "every Florida home" to be a center for "healthy, happy childhood."[74] The National Negro Health Week offered still another occasion. This program was initiated by Booker T. Washington, the principal of the Tuskegee Institute, and moved forward by his successor Robert Russa Moton to specifically engage African American communities across the South in health work.[75]

To be sure, African Americans in the health professions were poorly represented in Florida, as they were across the South. In their absence, National Negro Health Week was an opportunity for concerned African Americans as

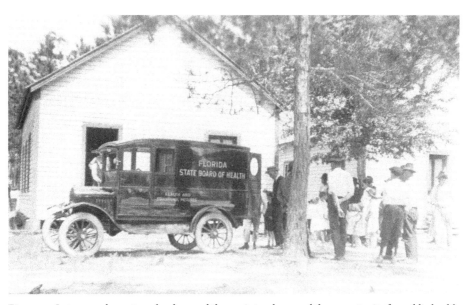

Figure 2.2. In town and country schools, a mobile movie truck opened the opportunity for public health nurses to engage with a wide range of residents, from city folk to those at farms, turpentine stills, and lumber mills. 1924. Courtesy of the State Library of Florida.

well as the State Board of Health to highlight the toll on African Americans of deaths from tuberculosis. In the mid-1920s Florida's count of deaths from the disease remained higher among African Americans than whites. In 1924 the state's population was approximately 66 percent white and 34 percent black, yet of a total of 1,054 deaths from tuberculosis, the number among African Americans was 579, far in excess of the deaths of whites, at 457.[76] During the week of daily programs, these stark figures drew doctors, public health nurses, social workers, ministers, and others in authority to lecture the community. "Health work has been found to be one of the most effective methods of bringing the two races together on a platform of mutual confidence and respect with a mutual desire to help," stated Robert Russa Moton, promoting National Negro Health Week throughout the South.[77] In April 1925, although only ten of Florida's sixty-seven counties observed the activities of National Negro Health Week, Reid took the credit for utilizing "all the nurses to stimulate health work among the colored people." Reid involved herself in the programs, offering assistance and forceful ways to drive the State Board of Health's message home as the information circulated. "Tuberculosis (consumption) is not

hereditary but is spread through carelessness; treatment should begin early,"
Florida Health Notes announced. "Aim for prevention: 1. Good cheer. 2. Good
food. 3. Fresh air. 4. Proper living."[78] Reid used the occasion as a springboard
to expand work. Reporting the nurses' activities to the Children's Bureau, she
noted, "Where ever possible health work of various kinds was conducted in
the Negro communities."[79]

Many lay African American women did not require a special event to place
health work into their own hands. Reid had only to look to Tampa to observe
work that exemplified Moton's platform. Many black women enrolled in the
American Red Cross Home Hygiene and Care of the Sick classes to care for the
ill at home and prevent the spread of tuberculosis and other diseases. In Tampa
the classes were taught by the Red Cross public health nurse Joyce Ely and once
again brought together the races in mutual understanding.[80] By 1924, 124 African American women had graduated from the Home Hygiene and Care of the
Sick classes of the Tampa chapter, indicating the program's success.[81] In 1928,
during the latter part of Reid's tenure, Ely joined Reid's team; in contrast to
Reid but in line with other colleagues, Ely evinced a less condescending manner toward midwives that more nearly followed Moton's "platform of mutual
confidence and respect."

By establishing links into Florida through local chapters, the American Red
Cross not only provided black and white women with home nursing classes but
also opened positions for professional black and white public health nurses.
The State Board of Health's employment of black nurses, however, remained
flat. Reid had expanded the state's public health nursing service and increased
the number of white state health nurses, but their race did not mirror the entire population they served. Only one black nurse, Estelle Bonner, remained
on the staff. Brandishing the slogan "Florida Nurses for Florida Work," Reid
had toured the state to visit hospitals and nurse training schools to enlist more
graduate nurses for public health work.[82] In 1925 she was a guest speaker at the
National Association of Colored Graduate Nurses convention held in Jacksonville, indicating her intention to increase the number of black state health
nurses.

This convention assembled Florida's prominent black graduate nurses to
participate in the ongoing national movement to advance their profession. Petra Pinn, the superintendent of Pine Ridge Hospital for ten years and fondly
dubbed "Mother Pinn" by the grateful residents, was the president who greeted
the nurse members from other states. Like Rosa Brown, who was also in at-

tendance, Pinn had taken an active leadership role in previous conventions of the organization. The movement had grown exponentially. At this Jacksonville convention Brown responded to the increasing interest and reported to the participants that there were two hundred membership inquiries nationwide and twenty-three applicants for membership. At this time there was no gesture of integration with either the national or state white associations. Thus, when a lengthy discussion ensued concerning whether to accept Bertha E. Deen, the white superintendent of Brewster Hospital, as a member, her application was refused.[83]

Other notable attendees included Bessie Hawes, who presided over the public part of the meeting. She was the president of the Jacksonville Local Nurses Association, an organization initiated by Rosa Brown in 1917 to unite the area's African American graduate nurses. Hawes had spent five years as a public health nurse in Palatka before relocating to Jacksonville for a position at the City Health Department. At the convention, Hagar H. Middleton, an African American Red Cross instructor, gave a presentation on her outreach to women and girls of her neighborhood with the Home Nursing and Care of the Sick classes. And the state health nurse Estelle Bonner's paper "Work among the Colored People In Florida" was very well received and led to a subsequent discussion about the "value of the midwife" that yielded "a great deal of valuable information." Laurie Jean Reid's address on "The Nurse and Her Work" received a polite rising vote of thanks. Reid "dwelt on the value of records," which proved to be a sermon to the converted, as many in the group were leaders of their nursing schools' alumni. The secretary's report underscored the point, indicating that Reid "enlarged on the following points—discussing shop worn articles, the value of study, keeping up one's ideals, respect for one's training school, respect for other people's property, kindness, lack of gossip and 'golden silence.'"[84] Yet if Reid had hopes of recruiting additional African American nurses for the State Board of Health, the decision to do so was taken out of her control.

Roadblocks and Red Cross Involvement

In 1926 the State Board of Health members determined that as a matter of policy only white nurses would be engaged as state health nurses.[85] Reid reported this policy to the Children's Bureau, writing about the forced resignation of the only African American employed by the State Board of Health, Estelle Bonner.

Reid complained to Abbott, "It has been difficult to explain the reason for a colored nurse on the staff to the satisfaction of the old conservative southerners in the state and it was finally decided to be the fixed policy of the State Board of Health not to employ negro nurses."[86] By eliminating Bonner's employment, the board ignored the reality that Bonner was an important conduit to connect Sheppard-Towner Act policies with African American people. Excluding the African American state health nurses hindered the state program but shone a light on the more inclusive Red Cross. Bonner continued work as a public health nurse for the St. Johns County chapter of the Red Cross in St. Augustine.[87] The new policy was a severe blow to Reid's program, but she maintained the theme of overcoming obstacles in spite of the crippling racial discrimination; she did not publicly announce that there was a racial barrier she could not defeat.

Further speculation about the firing incident warrants a suggestion that the state health nurse Ruth Mettinger objected to the board's racism. In October 1926, just two months after the state forced Bonner to resign, Mettinger resigned willingly. The more open policy of the Red Cross evidently appealed to her. She began work for the Red Cross of Winter Haven in Polk County, where she negotiated a way to bring African American nurses into Red Cross employment. "Although money has been tight all over the state, Miss Mettinger has managed to get the committee to see the importance of employing a colored nurse," wrote Charlotte Heilman (1880–1956), the Red Cross field representative. Heilman went on to praise Mettinger's collaboration with black and white nurses. She wrote that Mettinger "has shown rather unusual executive ability in her work in Winter Haven. She and the other white nurse [employed by the city] and the colored nurse are all working beautifully together and the others look to Miss Mettinger to the take lead." Heilman was so impressed with Mettinger's leadership that she considered Mettinger for a promotion as her replacement. Mettinger "would make a good field representative. . . . I have admired her determination to have the colored nurse and the office assistant and her ability to persuade the Chapter to employ them even though they did not know where the money was coming from."[88]

As the regional field supervisor, Mettinger saw her career accelerate with the Red Cross, but her personal dissatisfaction with state officials continued. "She does not trust them," one report revealed.[89] When Reid requested Mettinger's return to the Sheppard-Towner program as a field supervisor in 1928, Mettinger refused. "I like my work," Mettinger wrote, "and the people for whom I work and therefore I am perfectly satisfied with my present [Red Cross] position."[90] She conceded that she might consider dividing her time between the Red Cross and the State Board of Health, but she would only consider the option with caveats that again indicated her opposition to the state officials. "I hope it will not be until the first of the year," she wrote, "as at that time there will be a change in our governor and probably a change in State Board of Health Officials."[91] Reid was forced to concede that the promising trajectory of public health nursing she had created for the state was on a downward spiral compared to the apparent trajectory of the Red Cross Public Health Nursing Service.[92]

Reid was forced to take on a supporting role in public health initiatives when the Red Cross took the lead to respond to two catastrophic hurricanes two years apart, in 1926 and 1928, that devastated large areas of Dade and Broward Counties. The first hurricane, without a name, struck Miami on September 18, 1926. Almost 400 people died, and 18,000 families were affected by the storm. Two years later the September 16 West Indian hurricane struck Palm Beach County and the southeastern shore of Lake Okeechobee.[93] Approximately 2,000 people died, many of them seasonal laborers from the Bahamas. The Red Cross Nursing Service, built up with the intention of providing disaster relief, hastened to the scenes and set the well-oiled Red Cross machinery of disaster relief into action for both hurricanes.[94]

As the Red Cross rallied the in-state and out-of-state teams to deliver the emergency response, Reid made a point of publicizing that the state health nurses were well trained and at hand to provide immediate response for both hurricanes. In her final assessment of the nursing response, Reid glazed over the Red Cross involvement and instead utilized the disasters to once again promote the state health nurses' work. "Because we are a State Department, emergencies are common and looked upon as ordinary routine," she wrote for Florida Heath Notes. Every nurse drove her own car and was familiar with the area. "Since their regular work includes travel on roads in all kinds of weather and changes are part of their daily task, the storm-work was not so unusual for them it was just another task which was accomplished quietly and skillfully."[95] Reid reminded readers that it was the state health nurses who were the "proper" people to deliver relief. While her promotion of and pride in the state nurses' work spoke to the skill and practicality that the nurses brought to the emergency situation, hurricane relief was also an opportunity for Reid to drum into to the public the great advantages of the state nurses' work and at the same time promote her own leadership at a state level. In doing so she also distanced herself from the leadership of the Red Cross.

Privately, Reid's attitude toward the loss of life revealed once again her adherence to some important aspects of public health philosophy. After the first hurricane Reid wrote a personal letter to Grace Abbott, dated September 18, 1926, in which she directly expressed a viewpoint of eugenic theory: "In spite of the loss of life I do not consider the disaster an unmixed evil. From it must come a finer Florida and a finer people because the weaklings will have been weeded out."[96] While Reid sought her own answers for the devastating loss of life as well as the ill effects of changes in society, her response was a pessimistic outlook for the people of Florida.[97] Like Lavinia Dock, she was looking toward the science of eugenics to promote "developing a higher and nobler race of men," which Dock was convinced "must and will prove to be the most supreme and all-important all-embracing science known."[98] For Dock, Reid, and others, eugenics was the part of a movement aimed toward the betterment of the human condition.[99] Reid's statement "the weaklings will have been weeded out" was a reconfiguration of the view expressed in a 1912 nursing journal, that "natural selection rests upon excessive production and wholesale destruction; eugenics on bringing no more individuals into the world that can be properly cared for and those only of the best stock."[100] Reid's private opinion was at odds with her public statement that public health nurses "take in every suffering, helpless bit of humanity."[101] But not all of Florida's state health nurses evinced such beliefs.

Further Challenges for Reid

The promising trajectory of the public health nursing created by the Sheppard-Towner Act experienced a reversal in 1927 when the state decreased the appropriation for the state's public health nurses. Reid was forced to cut field staff. By 1927 the now thirteen public health nurses were reduced again to nine; five Sheppard-Towner nurses continued the work with maternal and infant hygiene, leaving four state-funded "rural school nurses" to address schoolchildren's health.[102] The void was obvious to I. Malinde Havey (1887–1938), the assistant director of the Red Cross Public Health Nursing Service. "Just how four nurses are to make themselves felt in this work is beyond me," she reported to the Red Cross headquarters after her visit to the state. "Of course they will confine themselves to communities that do not have any form of rural public health nursing work."[103] Reid likewise poured out her frustration with the lack of support from the state in *Florida Health Notes*. She wrote, "Unfortunately we are obliged, because of conditions and circumstances over which we have no control, to do our work with tools at hand, using our professional knowledge and ingenuity to attain the best results possible."[104]

At the same time, public health nursing links with the Red Cross had strengthened. In local communities where Red Cross public health nurses were replaced by their municipally funded counterparts, many nurses continued their connection with the Red Cross. If the "affiliation with the Red Cross is desired," noted Havey, "Mrs. Reid agreed that it should be granted."[105] Privately, of course, Reid did not desire it. There was an undercurrent of tension in the struggle for influence with the public health nurses of the state. Quick to pass judgment on Reid's character, Havey dismissed Reid as a "rough and ready somebody" and pointed out she was "frightfully jealous" of her assistant supervisor, Bertyne Anderson, "a cultured, well poised person with much personality and charm."[106] Havey admired Anderson, who was not only a state health nurse but also a clubwoman, the 1926 president of the now renamed Florida State Nurses Association, and the state chair of the Red Cross Nursing Service in Florida.[107] "I wish we might have her in our Red Cross official family for she is a most desirable person," Havey reported, hoping to recruit Anderson to a permanent position in the Red Cross Public Health Nursing Service.[108] Seemingly Anderson refused to be caught in the tug-of-war between Reid and the Red Cross and departed from the state. Reid was left to preserve the reduced number of state health nurses under her leadership. Her zeal to protect her position led Red Cross Field Supervisor Ruth Mettinger to conclude that Reid "more or less put a fence around her nurses and let no other bureau contact them or have any voice in the matter." For Mettinger, Reid's attitude was detrimental to establishing the roots of the profession in Florida. "It is too bad that one person can build up and yet destroy so much work in a state," she wrote.[109]

Reid's grappling with the Red Cross and the cutback in state health nurses coincided with the national struggle to continue with the appropriation for the Sheppard-Towner Act after it was scheduled to cease on June 30, 1927. Although many had considered it a permanent law, opponents renewed their 1921 opposition even more vehemently. The American Medical Association and other groups fought to reject a continuation of the act that they saw as a move to "socialize medicine" and "nationalize the children." The Women

Patriots group considered the women who led the whole progressive platform for children as "feminist-socialist-communist plotters." The Women Patriots influenced the Daughters of the American Republic to withdraw their support for extending the act. Eventually, the groups were forced to accept a compromise that extended appropriations only until June 30, 1929.[110] President Calvin Coolidge signed the extension into law on January 22, 1927. Reid appealed to her clubwomen allies to "share in this work . . . and see that the legislators from your county are familiar with the Act and the need for its continuance in order that Florida may be known as a state where mothers and babies are cared for as its most precious assets." Reid noted that while at first some of the more conservative clubwomen were unwilling to place the Sheppard-Towner nurses on their programs in their local clubs for fear of "what appeared to be, on the surface, something radical," those reluctant clubwomen joined their more forward-thinking peers and besieged Reid with requests for nurses to speak in their programs. Now Reid expected them to support the continuation of the act. As the extension of federal funding was contingent on the state legislature matching the funds, Reid demanded that the clubwomen turn out to lobby their representatives to vote for a continuance at its upcoming April session. "It is your share in this work," she lectured the clubwomen.[111]

By the time the Sheppard-Towner Act appropriation was discontinued in 1929, the number of midwives in Florida was reduced from 4,000 to 1,280. In fact, as Reid prepared to terminate her position, she noted that a "queer situation" had developed in the state. For seven years, public health nurses had been educating people to protect the lives of mothers and children. Communities and counties had grown "health conscious," Reid noted, "and now we find ourselves unable to give to the communities as large a service as they demand of us for lack of field personnel." Reid hoped that the State Board of Health could help arrange for the employment of suitable public health nurses in counties, organizations, or school boards. Meanwhile, she noted that the state would continue the Sheppard-Towner work with certain adjustments learned from "trials and triumphs" over the previous seven years. The midwife problem had begun its transition into the midwife program. Reid was adamant and declared, "The work with midwives must be continued if results are to remain satisfactory, since no other provision is made for their supervision."[112]

At the conclusion of the Sheppard-Towner Act program, the Bureau of Child Hygiene and Public Health Nursing had established a well-run, if inadequately staffed, headquarters aiming to cover the state with maternal and infant hygiene. The rural areas, however, remained sorely in need.[113] Reid acknowledged that though there remained an enormous gap between the services provided to urban and rural areas, the knowledge that public health nurses gained from their outreach to midwives and mothers would help to facilitate change. For Reid, the strength of the program lay not necessarily in the numbers of the public health nurses employed by the State Board of Health at that time but in the development of the public health nursing profession in Florida.

While she had established the leadership for county and community public health nurses from the board headquarters, she left only a small team of white state health nurses to continue the maternity and infant hygiene program in Florida, a record that compared poorly with its counterpart in Mississippi. By 1930 the Mississippi Board of Health had hired six black public health nurses to work alongside the 125 white ones.[114] Reid's frustration with Florida's racial policies finally surfaced publicly with her parting words of disdain to readers of *Florida Health Notes*: "All public health nursing should be based . . . on the following principles . . . an agency should be non-sectarian and non-political in spirit and service without distinction of race, creed or color."[115]

3

|||||||||||||||||||||||||||||||||||||||||||||||||||||||||||||||||||

Linking to Public Health Nursing
the Red Cross Way, 1919 to 1930

||||||||||||||||||||||||||||||||||||||||||||||||||||||||||||||||||||

"Have you ever thought of the Red Cross public health nurse as an artist?" asked Rosa Brown, writing in a November 1932 issue of the *Red Cross Courier*. She was reporting on her last three years' work as the Red Cross public health nurse for Palm Beach County and took the opportunity to expand upon a philosophy that had driven her cause from the early days of the founding of the National Association of Colored Graduate Nurses. "I like best to picture the nurse as the creator of great paintings with a brush that is her untiring service to suffering humanity," she wrote, "but it is my purpose to picture with very practical strokes a public health program for under privileged Negroes in a rural district."[1] Beginning in 1929 with a Ford car to cover 2,500 miles, Brown summed up the great strides she had made with her work, pointing out that her aim was "to help people help themselves and thus improve their condition physically, mentally and socially."[2] She was the only source to deliver public health intercessions that she reminded readers was as "basic to the general welfare of the Negro as to other races."[3] Public health officials, Red Cross representatives, and most importantly Brown herself evaluated her "practical strokes," her outreach, and her successes as exemplary.[4]

Brown took further action to detail her model work through a series of articles she wrote for the *Red Cross Courier* and the journal of the National Association of Colored Graduate Nurses as well as other African American publications.[5] Even the *American Journal of Nursing* acknowledged the value of her work but in a nod to ubiquitous racism published an alternative source.

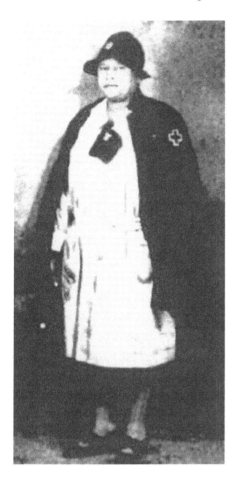

Figure 3.1. Rosa L. Brown served as a Red Cross nurse in Palm Beach County, 1929. From Frances Smith Dean, "Rosa L. Brown's Contribution to Her Own Race," *American Journal of Nursing* 31, no. 7 (July 1931): 841–842. Used with permission.

A writer for the *American Journal of Nursing*, Frances Smith Dean, conveyed the impression that Brown's work was incredible; the list of her achievements "reads like a fairy tale," she wrote. This account included the eloquent "brush strokes" of Brown's voice laying down the thesis that such work was indeed possible given the opportunity.[6] For Brown, her ground-breaking work was the realization of her longtime ambition that at last came to fruition. She seized the opportunity offered by the Red Cross to proceed with authority. She aimed to make sure her work mattered to those she termed the "less fortunate" of her race as well as to those who followed her path.

Brown's picture of the deplorable health conditions in Palm Beach County makes clear the absolute necessity of her work. "There are no health laws ob-served in the Negro section," she wrote, indicating that property owners bore a core responsibility for neglect. Brown's frank assessment heightened the contrast in the county between the neglected, downtrodden community and the modern, luxurious winter resorts on the coast that would be well known to health officials and many northern readers. "Anyone without question can build a row of stalls not nearly as sanitary as those built for well-bred horses," she wrote. "One family rents a stall 8 × 10, where they sleep or find room to sit down is a mathematical problem." If a pump was provided, there was no drainage, leaving wastewater to accumulate and become a rubbish dump and breeding place for mosquitoes, insects, and vermin. "Someday—I sincerely hope not in the far future—the white people in this section will learn, I trust before some dreadful disease invades their homes, that disease doesn't stay put," she stressed, picking up on the "germs know no color line" scare tactic utilized by both white and black health leaders.[7] Like Booker T. Washington when he founded National Negro Health Week, Brown spoke in blatant language to critique segregation and solicit action. The profound neglect of black communities' health was putting lives at risk.[8] But Brown was also aware that for those like Terry in Jacksonville it was a "matter of sheer self-preservation to the white man."[9] As the most vibrant advocate for black residents' health in her county, Brown concluded that "any one part of the community cannot be made safe while the other part is so badly neglected."[10] The work to improve conditions fell on her shoulders, and with no hesitation she spoke out loudly and drew in, as she put it, those "from the favorable race" who could assist her cause.[11]

Brown made it clear that the Red Cross, "that organization that mothers the world," deserved credit for its interest in initiating her public health work.[12] In Florida it was one of the few white organizations supporting health outreach into black communities, an endeavor that was even more critical given the State Board of Health's racial policies.[13] In 1929 Brown's work began as a Red Cross experiment that she ensured became permanent once she had proven the value of her work. Working out of her automobile, she built up the program gradually, adapting her work to fit the community. "Long before my professional day was supposed to begin the mothers and older children whom I sought to help would be out in the fields at work. My first step was to change my schedule to conform to their convenience," she noted.[14] In the evenings, she encouraged these working mothers to attend her Red Cross Home Hygiene and Care of the Sick classes. For the next step, she urged the women to participate in attaining community goals to improve conditions in their homes and communities. "The aim fixed was to help them to help themselves," she declared. She told of efforts to initiate a Home Beautiful campaign to turn a community around from a place where "wholesome recreation and community spirit were utterly lacking . . . [and] litter and unsightly weeds were the rule everywhere."[15] Twenty years earlier the Florida Federation of Women's Clubs had demanded that the common water dipper be abolished in white schools; now, in 1929, Brown initiated this fundamental reform in black schools.[16] Then she went on to establish a club for parents and teachers to support each other to uphold children's hygiene standards.[17] In a community that was so full of "hard work and anxiety," where people "knew nothing of the value of books and hygienic homes, because they were unable to read," Brown intended her health lessons and uplift in the community to save lives. Furthermore, she intended to solicit funds to provide recreational facilities and bring a "little light into the darkness and monotony of life."[18]

Confidently and firmly, Brown drew in supportive organizations by using the Red Cross name to pave the way for other philanthropic entities to contribute to health work in African American communities. After six months, at the end of the experiment, she had secured support to continue the program. The Kiwanis Club, Brown noted, was willing to provide for underprivileged children's health needs regardless of color. The club was essential to Brown's health program by facilitating hospitalizations and establishing dental and eye clinics for rural children. Her emphasis on preventive measures and instruction on social diseases and sanitation appealed to Joe Youngblood, the superintendent of public instruction in Palm Beach County, and F. E. Bryant, the vice president of Southern Sugar Corporation. Both pledged funds to the Red Cross chapter in Palm Beach County to supplement her work. Later, Dr. Henry Hanson, the state health officer, obtained support from the Julius Rosenwald Fund as well. Brown ensured that the Red Cross experiment became permanent. After more than two decades, she was finally fulfilling her vision, one shared by the National Association of Colored Graduate Nurses. "By slow degrees, the Negro nurse is doing her part to help develop her people," Brown asserted.[19] And just as Gantt found in 1916, the people, in turn, appreciated the public health nurse. "I found the colored people most cooperative," concluded Brown, "unselfish and loyal, ever ready to profit from health instruction."[20]

In 1926 Florida's State Board of Health had slammed the door firmly shut on its employment of black public health nurses, while the Red Cross kept the door open and Brown utilized its policy of accommodation to her advantage. For Brown, "The spirit and influence of the Red Cross had helped these people [benefactors] to grasp more clearly the meaning of the Good Samaritan." With broad brush strokes she painted a religious tone to her work that was central to her philosophy and the Red Cross mission as well. "As I see the Red Cross public health nurse," Brown intoned, "she is the practical application of the Great Physician[,] . . . not something beautiful beyond the clouds but heaven here on earth—a heaven of good health, clean bodies and minds, of better sanitation, of clean homes, and thus better citizens, a better community, a better State, a stronger and healthier nation."[21] Brown underscored the founding spirit of the Red Cross Nursing Service and wove it into her work. The American Red Cross Nursing Service "need not go back further than the Good Samaritan," wrote Lavinia Dock in her definitive 1922 book, *History of American Red Cross Nursing*. The originating principles of the Red Cross were based on "the spontaneous, voluntary helpfulness of the private citizen [and] compassion and aid extended freely on the sole ground of common humanity."[22] Such an underlying philosophy spoke directly to Brown's work. It was a philosophy that drove the Red Cross Nursing Service during World War I, nurtured public health nursing, and fostered outreach into Florida the Red Cross way.

After the war the Red Cross developed public health nursing throughout the nation, extending its reach into the neglected parts of the South including Florida. Although it facilitated Brown's work, it had taken a decade of Red Cross nursing activity in Florida before her experiment could take shape. Through the 1920s, Darlene Clark Hine has argued, the Red Cross continued to underutilize black nurses in the region.[23] The "mother of the world" was not colorblind; the issue of race and nurse recruitment hampered its own policies, as Brown and her fellow members of the National Association of Colored Graduate Nurses were fully aware.[24] To be sure, in Florida with so few opportunities for black public health nurses to find work, the Red Cross employed white nurses to fill the void of delivering health services to African American communities and rural areas, but Red Cross policy and southern custom limited their reach. The articulate Brown never missed a chance to remind people that the black nurse was ready for service where and when she was needed. "Edified and inspired by the more favored race she becomes inspired to carry the light of health and sanitation to the less fortunate members of her race," Brown reiterated.[25]

Rooting Red Cross Public Health Nursing in Black and White

The new focus on public health after World War I was a vision clearly delineated by Jane Delano, the director of the Red Cross Nursing Service. Before leaving for her inspection tour of nurses stationed in Europe, she insisted that "one of the first things in the peace program of the Red Cross will be the further development of public health nursing . . . even [in] the most remote parts of the country."[26] The Red Cross nurses had set the wheels in motion overseas in seeking to improve the health of citizens in the war-torn countries of Europe. They were an essential component to the rebuilding of Europe, bringing reforms in public health and nursing that, as Julia Irwin has noted, became an important part of US foreign policy even as they imparted "a level of cultural authority and coercive power."[27] After Delano died in 1919, Clara D. Noyes replaced her as the director and took over her initiatives. Noyes believed that the Red Cross nurses' work in Europe needed to be brought home. "Now that you have proven what you are capable of doing, *can you demobilize*?" she wrote to the Red Cross nurses. "Is not life here at home as precious as a life in France? Will you not carry on the Red Cross peace program in its fight against preventable disease?"[28] Evidently, Noyes was not addressing the recently recruited black Red Cross nurses. To their chagrin, not one of them was mobilized overseas; not one of them had that choice. Though the National Association of Colored Graduate Nurses had long moved to fulfill black nurses' desire to join the Red Cross, issues of race had plagued their acceptance and complicated their delivery of service, whether in war or peace.[29]

In April 1917, at the onset of the United States' entrance into World War I, Rosa Brown's fellow association members sought to change the status established in 1911 during the early days of the Red Cross organization, when black nurses were denied inclusion in the Red Cross Nursing Service. The service provided a ready team to respond to natural disasters, but as it was also the route into the Army Nurse Corps, the surgeon general's office declared that their race made them ineligible for inclusion, on the grounds "of the impossibility of securing proper quarters for them."[30] Initially the Red Cross enrolled 8,000 white nurses for service, but as the war progressed the Army Nurse Corps required many hundreds more. Jane Delano expected to enroll black nurses to serve the black troops at the base hospitals. Her appeal for "150 nurses to enter Red Cross work" was read out at the August 1917 convention of the National Association of Colored Graduate Nurses, prompting several communications between Delano and the association's president, Adah B. Thoms.[31] Delano promised that black nurses would have "all the privileges of the white nurses. . . . They will receive the same pay and allowances, as all other nurses," she wrote in a letter to Thoms.[32] Their assignments, however, depended on the surgeon general's decision. In December, Dora E. Thompson, the superintendent of the Army Nurse Corps, only agreed to tentative future plans: "I think it might be advisable to enroll them, as should the need arise later they would be available for service," she wrote to Delano.[33] Not until July 1918 did the first nurses enroll, but still the delay of their assignment to duty dragged on, prompting Delano to send a telegraph to the National Association of Colored Graduate Nurses convention to explain: "The Red Cross is blameless with the colored nurses not being utilized," she insisted.[34]

Finally, the grave influenza epidemic drove the decision to assign the African American Red Cross nurses. An emergency contingent of nine arrived at Camp Sherman, Ohio, in early December 1918, almost a month after Armistice Day. Others followed to Camp Grant, Illinois, and Camp Sevier, South Carolina. These nurses opened the path into the Red Cross Nursing Service, and as Mary Sarnecky, a historian of the US Army Nurse Corps has noted, they made a first step in the integration of the Army Nurse Corps.[35] But only a small number of the eighty-two black nurses who received the prestigious Red Cross badges between July 2 and December 1, 1918, were assigned to duty.[36] By 1920 only two black registered Red Cross nurses went on to bring the fight against preventable diseases to Florida.

If their struggle to gain acceptance into the Red Cross Nursing Service was not enough to mark their difference, the prestigious Red Cross badge clarified it. As of July 1909, each enrolled Red Cross nurses received a Red Cross pin with her name and number engraved on the back. Records of the names and numbers were kept on file at the headquarters in Washington, DC.[37] Once African American members joined in July 1918, on the back of the badge the Red Cross engraved the letter "A" after their names and the numbers to distinguish their race. Delano explained the policy to division directors, and it continued through 1949. All African American applicants, she wrote, "should be listed as colored, so that in enrollment there may be no possibility of assigning them to duty without reference to color."[38] Florida's two recent inductees, Susan Barks and Mary Allen, worked for Jacksonville's City Health Department, but Rosa Brown was not listed. By the time she took up her position for the Palm Beach Red Cross chapter in 1929 she was forty-five years old. Her officially filed title was "home defense nurse," though in practice she worked under the title of "county Red Cross nurse."[39]

Making a Start

During the postwar decade a few black Red Cross nurses joined the many white nurses who answered Noyes's call to transition from war nursing to focus on public health at home. Kimberly Jensen has argued that this new class of nurses would not accept the demobilization of women's power called for by the popular press and civic leaders. Many were not interested in a "postwar bargain" that offered patriarchal protection in exchange for reinstating their traditional roles as women. Most saw the opportunity to link their professional service to the nation with the fruits of citizenship including the vote and military rank for nurses.[40] Prior to her appointment as the state field nurse for the Florida Tuberculosis Association, the Red Cross nurse Ada M. Whyte showed a typical motivation. In her application to the burgeoning Red Cross Bureau of Public Health Nursing she wrote, "I should especially like some work that would necessitate my training. Nearly a year of moving about in France has made the thought of settling in one place rather difficult."[41] Florida would certainly satisfy her desire for mobility as she conducted segregated tuberculosis clinics from Pensacola to Miami and went on to become the Florida Tuberculosis Association's supervisor of nursing.[42] Single or married and whether they chose a dedicated career or remained on the reserve list to be at the ready to respond to national disasters and emergencies, the graduate nurses' alliance with the Red Cross offered a path to combine their professional training with patriotic and humanitarian service.[43] Florida was a fertile field to reap the benefits of their skill, as Whyte and Ruth Adamson, the regional field director for the Red Cross Bureau of Public Health Nursing, as well as other Red Cross nurses soon discovered.

Yet, through the 1920s the underpinnings of conflict between county and state health bureaucracies hampered the local development of public health services and made it difficult for the Red Cross to grow its outreach. From the State Board of Health's perspective, the district health officers adequately covered the state, and besides, state law forbade any financial support to local health programs that were not statewide endeavors. Although the board's district officers oversaw health practices in towns, they did not venture into the rural areas. Most rural communities remained bereft of any services whatsoever.[44] But even as the growth of the Red Cross chapters during the war opened a springboard to serve these areas with Red Cross nurses, the success was contingent upon the local groups accepting Red Cross standards of organization and administration.[45]

Jane Van de Vrede (1880–1972), the director of the Red Cross Southern Division, headquartered in Atlanta, declared that the difficulty in reaching people and increasing services throughout the South stemmed from local opposition.[46] "The Southern people are more ready to accept state policy in contradiction to one announced by a national body and there is a marked conservatism in accepting all innovations," she reported to the Washington, DC, headquarters. In Florida particularly, there was no state policy directed toward public health nursing for people to accept! Filling the void was exactly what Van de Vrede intended, but unlike what occurred with the more cooperative states of North Carolina, South Carolina, Tennessee, and Georgia, she could not reach either a formal or informal agreement with Florida's State Board of Health. She concluded that solving the overall problem amounted to establishing Red Cross standards in the minds of people including the health officials "of many hitherto unapproached and almost unapproachable localities" of Florida.[47]

One such locality was Palm Beach County, where tensions flared up between Van de Vrede and the powerful Joe L. Earman, the owner of the *Palm Beach Post* and the chairman of the State Board of Health.[48] The incident exemplified the difficulties of bringing national leadership into a local community where powerful citizens claimed the responsibility to direct the local response in health-related affairs.[49] Like most patriotic citizens, Earman supported the Red Cross during the war and saw the advantages of supporting the local Red Cross chapter to hire a Red Cross nurse. She was particularly needed in the neglected rural areas of Palm Beach County to reach patients with tuberculosis, address child and maternal health, and teach preventive measures. With great fanfare, Katherine Huff, hailed as a "brilliant young woman with overseas experience," arrived only to be caught in the middle of the clash.[50] The difficulty arose when Earman did not agree with the Red Cross policies. He expected the Red Cross to provide and finance a catch-all public health service that would enable the school board to divert the money appropriated for a school nurse and augment the salaries of underpaid teachers. Earman presumed to sway Van de Vrede to do his bidding.

Earman sought to undercut Van de Vrede's influence by pointedly noting that he had his position at the State Board of Health along with the power and influence of the *Palm Beach Post* at his disposal and could either assist or impede the Red Cross in its drives and work. Accordingly, he expected to provide leadership for Huff and the Red Cross to accede to his proposals. "HEALTH IS HEALTH," he wrote in capital letters, using his newspaper as a mouthpiece, "and there should be cooperation whereby results being sought by the Red Cross and the State Board of Health can be brought about." He bellowed that the local chapter at Palm Beach and especially the Red Cross nurse were not showing proper courtesy and cooperation.[51] Instead of backing down, Van de Vrede made it clear to Earman and Dr. Ralph N. Greene, the state health officer, that the Red Cross would cooperate with the board but did not intend to duplicate services or provide a free catch-all service.[52] In response, Earman hurled insults at Van de Vrede personally as well as at the Red Cross Nursing Service in general. "It seems that trouble makers are also in high places," he wrote. "I am constrained to state to you that the Department of Nursing of the Red Cross is more correspondence than efficiency." He insisted that he would be heard because as president of the State Board of Health he, not Greene, was the "head of the health of the state." Yet he finally backed down and attributed the controversy to the fact that he was dealing with women. To make his point clear he used capital letters: "There just AINT anyway to get a woman to do business according to business methods. . . . THEY DO JUST AS THEY PLEASE and all men can do is to SIT DOWN AND CUSS LOW UNDER HIS BREATH [*sic*]."[53]

With the backing of the Red Cross, Van de Vrede illustrated the growing power of women who did not support the so-called postwar bargain. Her status in the Red Cross gave her the authority to push gender and class boundaries, an assertiveness that Earman perceived as a threat and one that would feminize his domain of policy making and politics.[54] He saw Van de Vrede as a facilitator of national interference in local affairs, but Van de Vrede was not cowed by his authority. In fact, she dedicated her life to upholding Red Cross standards. Quite simply she revealed, "I can't live without the Red Cross. It's a part of me."[55] Although born in Wisconsin, Van de Vrede had built her career in the South first as a bacteriologist in Georgia and then in the Red Cross Nursing Service. She knew the South—the scattered centers of population throughout the region, the meager living conditions, the lack of good roads, the lack of appropriation for education, the poor schools, and the great health toll to both black and white rural people. She knew what a Red Cross public health service could bring. And she knew that Earman was in a position to back Red Cross public health work. Though Earman retreated from the skirmish, he was correct that the Red Cross needed his cooperation and that of other powerful community leaders in business and politics because the future of the Red Cross relied upon community support to elicit successful fund-raising campaigns, to finance the chapters, and to promote public health nursing.

The Black and White of Delivering Health Intercessions

After her first tour of Florida's field in November 1919, Ruth Adamson found that Earman's misunderstanding was typical. Several chapters lacked the understanding of the organization of Red Cross nursing activities, but she also found great possibilities for service if the nurses understood how the issue of race limited their reach. Her visit to Polk County, a "very prosperous and important agricultural county" in central Florida, brought the problem to light. This county had established three Red Cross chapters, but only one had managed to secure a nurse. Adamson noted the large "colored population" and the dire need of health education and nursing services to include follow-up visits to tubercular patients in their homes. Yet, in spite of the need, she reported that it was not feasible for white nurses to seek out people in their homes: "I find it is not desirable to have the white nurse do much house visiting among the colored people although educational work in schools and to groups of this race is quite permissible."[56]

Adamson went further to clarify a black nurse's secondary position within the chapter, making the point that "a colored nurse under the direction of a white nurse would always be welcome." Yet that concept raised problems too. In Daytona, one of the two chapters that she singled out as having at least some understanding of the organization of the Red Cross Nursing Service, she found that a black nurse "furnished" by the chapter to the Florida Tuberculosis Association was supervised by a white nurse without any public health nursing experience. The Florida Tuberculosis Association supplied several nurses under the direction of Ada Whyte to various communities for specific times to conduct clinics. The work included seeking out, following up, and reaching people at home, but Adamson found that people disregarded the Red Cross procedures. "No reports of the work have ever been sent to division and headquarters," complained Adamson. Adamson's insight demonstrated to Van de

Vrede that the essential sticking point to progress was education—of communities, of chapters, and of nurses, white as well as black. She saw the need to promote Red Cross scholarships to those black and white graduate nurses deficient in postgraduate public health courses. As Adamson had clarified that race dictated service in homes, Van de Vrede took action to work with the National Association of Colored Graduate Nurses to upgrade black nursing schools in the South and open opportunities for more black women to serve their communities.[57]

An opportunity for Van De Vrede to speak publicly about the void of services to African American homes came in October 1920 at the Southern Tuberculosis Conference held in Jacksonville. "We have been slow to adopt [a peace program] for our own near neighbors, the Negroes," she announced at the "Negro Session" of the conference."[58] The need was acute. She presented statistics for the South showing that the general tuberculosis death rate for African Americans was more than two and a half times higher than the rate among whites. African American women had twice as many miscarriages as white women, and twice as many African American babies as white babies died in their first year. Infectious diseases were almost one and a half times as frequent in American Americans than whites, and this, Van de Vrede pointed out, was preventable. The need for infant welfare, maternity, school, and general public health nursing was evident, but while she charted the usefulness a public health nurse could bring to the community, she also listed the setbacks along the way to achieving those goals. The great need for additional and upgraded training schools for black nurses as well as postgraduate public health training was an aim called for by the National Association of Colored Graduate Nurses. As the chair of the Membership Committee, Rosa Brown not only surveyed applicants but also toured hospitals throughout the South. She confirmed that several hospitals did not offer theoretical work and only "use the colored nurses as practical workers in the wards."[59] Van de Vrede soon called for meetings with the black leaders to address concerns.[60] Most immediately, however, she urged nursing employers "to annex" black nurses to their staff and concluded that two cities in Florida, Jacksonville and Orlando, had joined others of the South to sprout an "excellent beginning" to the launching of public health work.

Speaking to the African American participants of the conference, Van de Vrede affirmed that the "greatest part of the work will fall upon the colored people themselves" to raise funds and to support public health nurses in their neighborhoods.[61] She called for support of the African American societies, lodges, and the National Health Circle for Colored People. The circle, developed from a relief organization to serve African American soldiers and their families during the war, reorganized in 1919 to focus on African Americans living in neglected districts of the South. One of the most neglected was Palatka, a small, isolated lumber town in rural Putnam County, Florida.

Bessie Hawes (1892–1983), a Tuskegee graduate with postgraduate training became the circle's first appointee and the first public health nurse in the town.[62] Her interest in public health work arose from her work during the influenza epidemic after her graduation in 1918. Accompanying a doctor to visit a family in a remote area of Alabama, she found the mother and four children dead and four others very ill. Hawes stayed to care for the family. "For eight days and nights I did twenty-four hour duty never once lying down to rest," she recorded. "In fact, there was no place to rest, and then, I was too interested in my patients' recovery to attempt to sleep."[63] The circle facilitated Hawes's postgraduate public health training at Lincoln Hospital, and in 1920 she brought the new concept of community nursing to Palatka. According to Adah Thoms, though Hawes faced opposition from the town's leaders at first, she won them over with her general program of community work. Mothers clubs, health lectures, home visits, and even parades where she dressed girls like nurses paved the way to establish a health center to initiate a new concept of health care to a previously unserved community.[64]

Van de Vrede and her audience would appreciate the promise of Hawes's headway in this small, rural town as well as the potential for other cities and towns to follow the lead made by Jacksonville and Orlando. Jacksonville set the precedent in Florida when the African American community collaborated with the city's strong health department, founded the Colored Health Improvement Association, and spurred the employment of the first black nurses. Orlando, nestled in central Orange County, was the second city saluted by Van de Vrede. It boasted a social service department that the local chamber of commerce claimed was the "best and most complete" in Florida.

In Orlando, two white county nurses worked alongside Katura B. Taylor (1891–1966), the black public health nurse who was in charge of reaching African American children throughout the county. She was in the audience to hear Van de Vrede single out her department. She had a part in the work to ensure that all schoolchildren received regular physical inspections and follow-up care. If parents were unable to afford treatments, community action facilitated free medical and dental care and hospitalizations. Van de Vrede applauded this strong beginning in Florida and supported Taylor to receive a Red Cross scholarship and attend a tuberculosis course at Vanderbilt University prior to a postgraduate course at the Columbia University summer school.[65] Van de Vrede's promotion of public health work through the Red Cross and her steps to improve the educational standards of all nurses to better meet the health needs of all people underscored Robert Russa Moton's contention once again that mutual concerns in health work brought the races together.

Steady Growth in Chapters and Nurses

If health work was an opportunity to bring the races together, there were limitations. Adamson made clear that the only way the Red Cross Nursing Service could expand and effectively reach people to improve health was to ensure that nurses did not disturb the relations between races, sexes, or classes. One efficient way was through the Home Hygiene and Care of the Sick Classes designed to teach women and girls of both races how best to combat contagion, improve the health of the family, and treat people at home. In Florida the numbers of chapters inaugurating a public health nursing service began to increase, from four in 1920 to twelve in 1924, but not all included home hygiene classes.[66] Van de Vrede answered such a spotty response by engaging the Red Cross nurse Joyce V. Ely (1889–1979) as the itinerant home hygiene field instructor. She was the ideal candidate. After demobilization from the Army Nurse Corps, she attended a postgraduate course at Teachers College, Columbia University, to teach at nursing schools. With one year of instructor experience at St. Luke's Hospital School of Nursing in St Louis, Missouri, her alma mater, she was ready to employ her skills once again for the Red Cross.[67]

On March 22, 1923, news reached Tampa that "Miss Joyce Ely representing the nursing department of the American Red Cross . . . began working with a large group of negro women." The news quickly proliferated.[68] Tampa had one of the strongest Red Cross chapters in Florida, with the executive secretary, Ruth Atkinson, standing out for her collaboration with the African American community and support of the Booker T. Washington Branch of the chapter. She spearheaded a Home Service Committee in the newly founded branch to facilitate visits to African American ex-servicemen and their families and then to purchase a cemetery for Florida's African American war veterans. She saw the advantages the home hygiene classes could bring to the community.

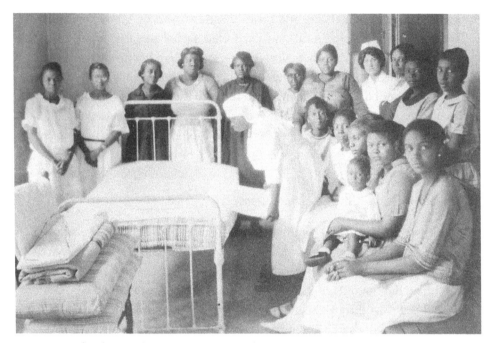

Figure 3.2. Ruth Atkinson, the executive secretary of Tampa's Red Cross chapter, observes bed making during a Home Hygiene and Care of the Sick class for the chapter's Booker T. Washington branch, 1923. Courtesy of the American National Red Cross Collection, Library of Congress.

With Negro Health Week of 1923 approaching, she drew on statistics provided by *The Negro Year Book* to encourage support for the classes: fifty out of every one hundred cases of illness could be prevented, and the annual loss of earnings from sickness and death could be reduced through knowledge of sanitation and hygiene.[69] Atkinson's experience as a fieldworker in the South gave her ready contact with Van de Vrede to coordinate Ely's arrival with the large group of enthusiastic black women enrolled by the Booker T. Washington Branch. Trumpeting the merits for the *Tampa Tribune*, Atkinson expected the fifty-five women graduating from the first set of classes to make "splendid practical nurses . . . [and] have a great influence on the health of Tampa."[70] The following year 124 women graduated from the home hygiene classes. The increased enrollment further rewarded Atkinson for her promotion of the health work in the black community.[71]

Joyce Ely began her public health career in Florida with the success of the home hygiene classes in Tampa. Van de Vrede recognized her ability to use the classes as a springboard to engage the community and assigned her to her next position, in Perry, a logging town in north Florida.[72] The Burton-Swartz Cypress Company, the largest producer of turpentine in the country, developed the town, employed most of the black and white residents, and supported them with company-owned houses, a drugstore, a doctor, and in 1923, a public health nurse. Ely remembered that on the day she arrived, flags waved and a band marched when the town turned out to greet her, including the president of the company and the mayor.[73] The overzealous greeting masked the underlying racial tension present in north Florida's rural communities.

From the white elite perspectives, the turnout to greet Ely served to reassure her of the influential white legacy of Taylor County and the corresponding white patriarchal duty to protect white womanhood. A few months prior to her arrival, in December 1922, the murder of a white schoolteacher in Perry led to a brutal trail of revenge. The attack against the white woman was an excuse for a lynch mob to react. In this case, the mob dragged the perceived culprit from jail to be burned at the stake, but one death was not enough. The mob ensured others, too, were lynched, and still others in Perry, beyond Taylor County, and over the state border into Georgia suffered the consequences of the white woman's murder. African Americans were left to rebuild burned-out homes, schools, and other property in the wake of the mob's terror.[74] One month later, Rosewood, a rural logging town in nearby Levy County, was the site of yet another racially motivated massacre. The events highlight the underlying smoldering tensions between the races and the triggers that sparked the brutal outbursts. This was the backdrop to the environment of Ely's new home. The schoolteacher was attacked on a road between the school and her home. Ely received a car and a house with a maid. If she was to address the health needs of both races within the company without disturbing the relations between the races, the home hygiene classes were an effective means. Fresh from the success of her classes in Tampa, Ely intended to expand her program carefully.

Ely's skills in communication and teaching helped her to make personal contacts with the company's women and those clubwomen in town without making home visits. According to Van de Vrede, the classes led to more cooperation and allowed the operation of more effective clinics. Ely "planned her program very definitely in the beginning to consider school work and classes with the mothers throughout the county in Home Hygiene and Care of the Sick." Crediting her as "one of the most successful nurses we have in Florida,"

Van de Vrede concluded, "we [at southern headquarters] feel that without the class work it would have been impossible to have the personal contacts and the work in many instances would have been more limited."[75]

During the 1920s, while the Sheppard-Towner nurses of the State Board of Health made inroads into maternal and child health, the American Red Cross Home Hygiene and Care of the Sick classes by growing numbers of Red Cross chapters became one of the most important methods of outreach. The classes remained constant programs even as the financial stability of the chapters varied and as some counties and cities took over public health nursing activities during the decade. Reporting monthly on nursing activities conducted by Florida's chapters, Charlotte Heilman, who took over Adamson's place as the nursing field representative, brought insight into the changing environment where the Red Cross opened opportunities for Red Cross nurses to slide into city or county positions.

The Tampa chapter exemplified the successful start with the home hygiene classes that led to the appointment of Madelyn Norton, "our colored nurse," who returned from a postgraduate class at Columbia University and planned to take her home hygiene classes into schools. She was, however, the last nurse on the chapter's payroll, continuing instead with the City Health Department. Along with Mary Potter, a white nurse, Norton intended to continue the classes and even develop first aid classes utilizing Red Cross material. In another example, during February 1927 the nursing program at the Lakeland chapter was taken over by the City Health Department, but the Red Cross nurse continued her classes in the high school. Then on one occasion the Red Cross facilitated an opportunity for a state nurse to transition to a chapter. After Estelle Bonner's dismissal from the State Board of Health solely on the grounds of her race, she began work for the St. Johns Chapter in St. Augustine, taking her classes into the industrial school. She joined Hagar H. Middleton, another African American nurse, who spoke about the home hygiene classes from an instructor's point of view to the nurse members of the National Association of Colored Graduate Nurses during its 1925 convention in Jacksonville.[76]

If the key to the effectiveness of the classes was the instructors' certain aggressiveness necessary to hold the interest of older women and school-age students from the community, the classes empowered all parties. Red Cross leadership held the classes to acclaim, noting the chapters conducting them and often singling out the nurse instructors. For the instructors the classes were a means to fulfill philosophical and practical goals. For the students, learning the skills of home nursing was a means to take responsibility for the health and well-being of themselves, their families, and their communities.[77] By 1930, fifty-five Red Cross chapters served Florida's rural and urban areas, with fifteen of them supporting public health nursing practices and eighteen conducting home hygiene classes. From Pensacola to New Smyrna, Jacksonville, Tampa, and Miami, white and black nurses recognized the value of the classes as a means to bridge the gap between modern health practices and the communities.

Hurricane Relief and Public Health Outreach

In 1926 and 1928, when two severe hurricanes devastated south Florida, the nursing response illustrated how far the professional, systemized Red Cross Nursing Service had come since its founding in 1910. It was after her service during Jacksonville's yellow fever epidemic that Jane Delano envisioned a ready supply of trained professional nurses to respond to disasters and took steps to build up a reserve.[78] After its exemplary service during World War I and public health work in the war's aftermath, the Red Cross Nursing Service was at the ready to respond to the nation's disasters including Florida's hurricanes. News of the first hurricane unleashed the chain of command from Red Cross headquarters to direct the relief funds including the Red Cross reserve nurses who would respond to the emergencies. Nurses were the key people to administer aid in the storm's aftermath, declared Clara Noyes, explaining that they "have the actual picture of what was done."[79] The well-oiled machinery of Red Cross hurricane relief work proved particularly effective in Florida due to the force of prepared nurses and their focus on public health outreach particularly in the flooded rural areas.[80]

Bertyne C. Anderson, a state health nurse, the state chair of the Red Cross Nursing Service of Florida and president of the Florida State Nurses Association ("Graduate" had been dropped from the association's name), was well situated to demonstrate how the dynamic relationship between the reserve rank of Red Cross nurses and the state health nurses strengthened the nursing response. They shared a self-proclaimed moral obligation to allay suffering. Like many others, it was the prospect of alleviating suffering during the war that drew Anderson to the Red Cross in the first place. "I feel I should get into this and do what I can," she wrote from her Jacksonville home when first applying for the nursing service.[81] After continuing her service in Greece and

Turkey after the war she demobilized to Florida, arriving at the State Board of Health in 1924 and quickly assuming leadership positions to see what she could do for Florida. Before the hurricane hit she had ensured that Florida's reserve Red Cross nurses were kept abreast of policy and were at the ready to meet any emergency.[82]

The hurricane that began as a tropical storm in the Atlantic made landfall near Miami on the evening of September 18, 1926, followed by eleven hours of fear and panic for 300,000 people in south Florida. At its peak, winds reached 138 miles per hour. A tidal wave washed over Miami Beach, and the surge pushed the Miami River over its banks and flooded the streets. Buildings collapsed and power lines were destroyed. After devastating the Miami area, the hurricane moved northwest to flatten the levee at the south end of Lake Okeechobee. Moore Haven was wiped out, and five other small farming towns were devastated. The hurricane brought havoc to more than fifty square miles of territory in Dade, Broward, and Palm Beach Counties.[83]

News reached Red Cross headquarters in the early hours of Sunday, September 19, initiating the Red Cross nursing response. Top-down national leadership began with Olive Chapman, a Red Cross public health nursing leader with experience in disaster relief after the tristate disaster in March 1925 when a deadly tornado swept through Missouri, Illinois, and parts of Indiana. Coming from Colorado, Chapman arrived in Miami by September 21, 1926, to open the American Red Cross disaster headquarters and coordinate those called to service. Anderson had sent wires to Florida's local Red Cross committees to call into action those nurses they had "line[d] up . . . in readiness."[84] Charlotte Heilman, the nursing field supervisor for Florida, cut short her vacation in Maryland. Jane Van de Vrede came from Georgia. Some local reserve nurses like Gertrude Rubelli lost their homes in the storm but still "served day and night until relieved by those called in from other places."[85] Approximately 350 Red Cross nurses arrived for duty including five African American nurses. One was Rosa Brown, and others were "loaned by the Negro Branch of the East Volusia Chapter A.R.C." All were graduate nurses. Chapman singled out the black nurses to recognize their "very helpful contribution to the work among their own group."[86]

Chapman directed efforts from Miami, assigning nurses to staff the temporary hospitals and emergency relief stations opened in various parts of Miami. Mary G. Fraser, the Red Cross supervisor of nurses in Dade County, assisted as a liaison between Chapman and local health authorities. Prompt action enabled approximately 30,000 people to receive the first inoculations of typhoid serum.[87] Fraser handled requests for relief and information about missing relatives from the hardest-hit areas, particularly Hialeah. Many homes were left in shambles and lives devastated; among those hit hard were some residents of Miami's tourist camps when the storm destroyed their flimsy, canvas shelters. Chapman placed a large unit of Red Cross nurses to visit the camps three times a day in a quest to avert disease. The "very undesirable quarters," Fraser reported, "are breeding places for all types of disease."[88] With Miami adequately covered, Chapman turned to Laurie Jean Reid to help avert the outbreak of disease in the devastated areas to the north up to Pompano, particularly those that were hard to access in the rural backcountry.

The backcountry and the devastated areas north of Miami to Pompano included the flooded towns around Lake Okeechobee, areas familiar to Reid and the state health nurses. On her initial survey of Moore Haven, Clewiston, South Bay, Belle Glade, and other devastated areas around Lake Okeechobee,

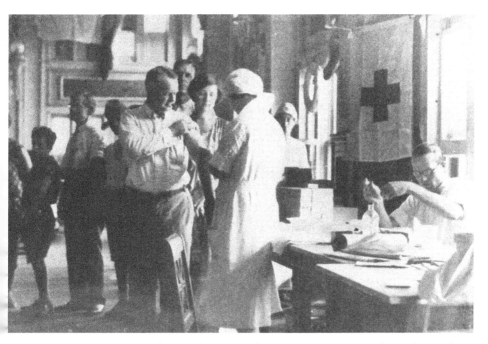

Figure 3.3. A nurse vaccinates people at a Red Cross inoculation station in a temporary hospital at McAllister Hotel in Miami after the 1926 hurricane. Courtesy of the Arva Moore Parks Photographic Collection.

Reid reported severe floods and many deaths. At Moore Haven "they took out of two feet of water 56 whites and 46 colored bodies," she noted. At Clewiston people had evacuated and the surrounding farmland was a "blank under 11 feet of water." At South Bay one woman was sent to hospital, but no one was killed. Belle Glade suffered the highest loss, with 611 dead, and those who remained faced food shortages. Stopping at every place on her way from West Palm Beach, Reid assessed the situation. The backcountry near Delray was in "great need for public health nurses to make a check of the territory." While the state health nurses were hurrying to the scenes in their cars, in Fort Lauderdale, Bertyne Anderson, the "capable Red Cross nurse with the State Board of Health," was ready to see what she could do at her temporary headquarters in the Masonic Temple. According to Reid, Anderson was most needed as "politics and mix-ups" prompted eleven Chicago nurses to leave, saying they would not be back.[89]

Reid maintained that the state health nurses were trained to provide prophylaxis and had the necessary skills to organize the district Red Cross Relief stations.[90] Other Red Cross nurses and a few doctors joined them to administer immunizations, provide dressings, distribute clothing, and accelerate transportation. Conducting surveys of the territory, visiting homes, and interviewing families, however, was left to Jule Graves, Beulah Heiber, Clio McLaughlin, Laura Niblock, and other state health nurses.[91] Many people left the flooded areas. At Sebring and Moore Haven, Jule Graves and Beulah Heiber worked around the clock to transfer refugees onto relief trains. Clio McLaughlin, covering the backcountry of Davie, illuminated the difficulties of enticing people to comply with disease prevention. She noted that families remaining in the backcountry had to be closely observed: "Sanitary needs must needs be watched, if we are to prevent disease." Many did not come forward to be immunized, and prophylaxis was slow, but "no attempt was made to induce people to be immunized until the nurses began their survey in the community."[92] McLaughlin's report demonstrates the vital role a public health nurse played as a bridge to induce people to receive immunizations. Laura Niblock, too, reporting from Glades County, revealed the difficulty to reach people physically and get the importance of prophylaxis through to them. "This district was conducted from the lake side since water made it impossible to get to all the points from land," she noted.[93] Meeting the needs of the Glades people was particularly challenging. "The Glades people will not accept anything from anyone unless need is imperative and must be watched to prevent suffering later," Niblock reported.[94] Even though much of the area in the district was flooded or waterlogged, Reid reported, nurses reached 221 homes and surveyed 284 families. But she also warned that as soon as the water was down, careful supervision would be important, as there were many babies and children in the area. "If we would maintain the health of these children much instructive work must be done," she asserted.[95]

Surveys of the various areas were completed by October 15; exceptions were those areas in South Bay and Chosen where the water had not receded. The small towns in the storm-hit areas were slowly recovering; by the end of October the entire district was free of communicable disease. People were depending less on area stations for care each day; thus, the district stations no longer required the large staff of nurses. Most of the state health nurses returned to their former duties. Reid reported that the state health nurses had visited pregnant women and people with injuries, instructed families about sanitary measures, and searched for signs of communicable diseases. The ongoing difficulty of reaching the Glades people, however, remained.[96]

The collaboration between the Red Cross and the State Board of Health nurses resulted in the sheer number of professionally trained women performing unique work. Doctors were not in such great demand following the immediate emergency. While there were 341 Red Cross nurses employed for the relief effort, the Red Cross employed only five physicians from September 21 to October 2, 1926. To avert criticism, Dr. William R. Redden, the Red Cross medical adviser, sent for twenty-six more doctors, even though they were not needed. He reported, "It was almost impossible to find enough work to keep them busy. In fact, at least ten of the group returned to their homes immediately. The remainder . . . gave effective service at tourist camps and some of the inoculation and dressing stations."[97] Redden's report underscores how far the Red Cross Nursing Service had come; the nurses were the backbone of preventive care and the most suited to reach out to families and avert suffering.

The 1928 Hurricane, Collaboration, and Service

When the September 1928 hurricane hit Puerto Rico, the Virgin Islands, and Florida, the Red Cross Nursing Service was once again set in motion. Elizabeth Fox, the director of Red Cross Bureau of Public Health Nursing, arrived in

Florida. Ruth Mettinger, now the field representative for Florida and Georgia, was close at hand to assist Fox.[98] Laurie Jean Reid and the team of state nurses immediately prepared to help. She declared that a public health nurse was the "proper person" to meet the needs of the flooded community. Drawing on her experience from the 1926 hurricane, once again she pointed out that a public health nurse would be aware of the continual problem with people who failed to comply with prophylaxis. "Lay people do not always put the proper value on small wounds and the need for immunization," she wrote. And raising the public health nurse's status above that of a private-duty or hospital nurse, Reid made it clear that "from her contact with people in their homes [the public health nurse] has a better background in instructive work."[99]

The devastation around Lake Okeechobee during the 1926 hurricane paled in comparison to the enormous toll in human lives caused by the hurricane of 1928. The storm destroyed the dike protecting South Bay, Belle Glade, Chosen, Pahokee, Miami Locks, and other small communities near Lake Okeechobee.[100] Many West Indian, Bahamian, and other laborers lost their lives. The official death toll mounted to 1,836.[101] The probable toll was far higher.[102] The post-hurricane relief effort, however, was marked by race, as Stuart Schwartz has noted. He examined the role of the Red Cross reconstruction policy and the influence of local leaders to focus relief on the more prosperous towns of Delray and Pompano rather than the poor farming communities where so many migrant workers lost their lives.[103] It was these poor rural communities that once again highlighted the joint effort between the Red Cross Nursing Service and the state health nurses to prevent and alleviate suffering in the unserved and underserved areas.

During the first two weeks, Elizabeth Fox, Reid, and other nurses worked with the backdrop of the National Guard, the Red Cross, and volunteers' efforts to focus immediately on hauling the drowned bodies and dead animals from the floodwaters and muck, burying and disposing of the often decomposed bodies and carcasses, and coping with the refugee transportation out of the area.[104] The state health nurse Jule Graves captured the horror of the situation in two versions of her narrative many years after the event. She intended to place it with a collection of her experiences in a book of her Florida stories, but she mistook the date. In one note headed "In Sept. 1933 when a hurricane was brewing," she described her call to action by "Laurie Jean Reid, Director of Bureau of P.H.N." Reid had left the bureau in January 1930, but it seems that for Graves the date faded to the background of the subject matter. As oral historians reiterate, it was the process of recalling her individual experience within the social context that allowed her to make sense of the past.[105] The actual date was not significant to her at all; what mattered was the tragic loss of life.[106] Graves described the stormy conditions of her journey from Live Oak, where she received Reid's call, to hurry to the hurricane headquarters at West Palm Beach. Her accounts stand out for the graphic content of her description of the subsequent loss of life that she found when she finally made it to her destination at Canal Point.[107] Graves recalled, "Local people joined into a death squad to find dead bodies . . . [and] people trying to find their dear ones. One man had his two little boys holding each one by the hand and a big wave took one of the boys. So the father was trying to find him."[108] Without sentimentalizing about the drowned bodies Graves discovered in the floodwater, she conveyed the horror of the disaster.

With such a large number of dead, Fox did not need the great influx of Red Cross nurses from other states that was necessary in 1926. She reported that the inoculation program was heavy but manageable. "We have not called upon those outside the state except for Savannah, Georgia, because we have been able to get nurses as needed to scene of action," she wrote.[109] And as in the aftermath of the 1926 hurricane, Fox drew upon the state health nurses to assume responsibility for the outlying districts. Jule Graves, Laura Niblock, and Clio McLaughlin had also worked through the 1926 hurricane and supervised the immunization programs in the backcountry.[110] The number of injured who required care was also manageable. White and black Red Cross nurses cared for the victims, separated by race, in segregated tent hospitals. Fox reported, "We have not had very many serious injuries, not much sickness. I think total of our hospital cases has been about 250[,] . . . some of them with serious fractures or with pneumonia or other acute conditions."[111] Fox's problems centered on the administration and accounting of hospital admissions.

The issue of hospital admissions added to the complaints local officials piled on the Red Cross. Fox demanded a dividing line between those "with a doubtful claim to a disaster-connected-illness and those who were sick previous to the disaster, but who met losses and cannot pay for medical care." Fox explained, "We are finding it most difficult to draw a line between proper Red Cross charges and those that are not." The Red Cross would only provide hospital admission for hurricane-related injuries and illnesses. Her solution was to arrange for three Red Cross nurses to investigate those cases still at home and waiting for hospital admission.[112]

The West Palm Beach commissioner complained that he had received many criticisms of the Red Cross's "alleged inefficiency" and called for the organization to "open its books." Ruth Mettinger tried to ease the situation as a bridge between the Red Cross and the local elites who had complained about the denial of hospital admissions. She was met with a slanderous attack on the Red Cross and the Red Cross nurses. That person, Mettinger reported, "stated I was a crook, the same as all the other Red Cross workers, keeping the money [to] dine at the finest hotels and receive exorbitant salaries, that the poor patients . . . were deprived of the cream off their milk in order nurses may use it."[113] The attack on the Red Cross was similar to the altercation between Joe Earman and Jane Van de Vrede in that powerful community members expected the Red Cross to fund a catch-all service for the poor. Mettinger's failure to ease tensions illustrated the problem of administering a top-down service to a local community where officials were quick to criticize an outside force even if it was providing a humanitarian service. The incident also highlights the challenges of the enormous accounting detail that hampered the Red Cross nurses from providing service to all the hurricane victims.[114]

Rosa Brown's New Path

As Ruth Mettinger began to close down the Red Cross Nursing Service hurricane relief activities by December 22, 1928, she arranged for Rosa Brown to be kept on the disaster payroll for one week longer.[115] Brown had stood out as an exemplary nurse at an African American tent city. "She has done a great deal toward promoting the Red Cross among her people and creating a friendly feeling," Mettinger reported.[116] Fox agreed. "Keep Nurse Brown on as long as you need her," she suggested.[117] As the Red Cross relief effort wound down, the Red Cross leadership saw Brown as a conduit to channel Red Cross public health nursing services to the unserved black communities of West Palm Beach. Her service would fulfill the Red Cross goal of providing "intelligent, indispensable service to a community . . . [that] necessitates *understanding* of what a community needs of its resources, as well as a wise linking up of program and resources cooperatively with other local organizations."[118] In this case, the wise linking up was between Rosa Brown and the Palm Beach Red Cross chapter. The direct result of Brown's work in the black tent city became what Brown called a Red Cross "experiment that led to permanency."[119]

In Florida the short-term disaster relief contributed to the foundation for long-term health work and disease prevention by public health nurses like Rosa Brown. Their work had lasting effects on communities, as the public health historian John Duffy has noted. He argues that the Red Cross is well known for its work during catastrophes and emergencies, but local public health work was also fundamental in providing health education leading to the formation of local county health units.[120] The Red Cross nurses worked in collaboration with the State Board of Health and Laurie Jean Reid, the state's director of public health nursing. Their work was contingent upon a team of well-qualified nurses to build up the profession. Working side by side or in complementary roles, they adapted their work to prevail over cultural and environmental obstacles. The need for such work in the aftermath of the hurricanes shone a national spotlight on the state's particular and vulnerable location.

4

|||||||||||||||||||||||||||||||||||||||||||||||||||||||||||||||||||||||||||||

Reaching Out to Midwives and
Country People, 1930 to 1947

|||||||||||||||||||||||||||||||||||||||||||||||||||||||||||||||||||||||||||||

It is largely due to Jule O. Graves, who transitioned Florida's "midwife problem" into the State Board of Health's "midwife program" and went on to lead
it from 1935 to 1947, that accounts have survived to offer insights into and
nuances of the relations between the nurses, midwives, and country folk.
Her photographs, often with short descriptions scrawled on the back, the
notes of her experiences in the field that she intended to turn into a book of
Florida stories, and the data collected from midwives including superstitions
and folk beliefs, along with her formal accounts and reports, offer a wealth
of firsthand material.[1] In one photograph, for example, Graves used her pen
to capture an African American midwife's voice to narrate the midwife's perspective of deep-seated troubles. This midwife attended a mother wedded
to folk beliefs that not only caused problems for the midwife but went on to
risk the life of the infant.

> Broward Co. midwife had been taught by the "bode" [State Board of
> Health] that the bed and not on the floor or on her "ol man's lap" was
> the place to deliver patients. She also knew that the baby's cord was her
> responsibility. A Nassau woman had given her trouble, saying both of her
> children had been born on the floor. The midwife finally delivered her
> on the bed. Before going home next day the family was warned not to let
> anyone touch the baby's cord dressing. When the midwife looked at the
> cord dressing on her return, she found that it had been "pranked" with

a "black lookin mess" (probably axel grease and soot) added. This was the last straw and the outraged midwife sent for the nearest State Health Officer and told him her troubles. He was reported to have 'cussed dem people comin an' tol dem he'd put every man Jack of dem in jail if he heard another word of complaint from the midwife.[2]

On one level Graves may have intended her record to serve multiple purposes. First, it absolved the midwife from possible repercussions of the dangerous practice. Second, it demonstrated the effectiveness of the midwives' training. Third, it illustrated the board's backup to the midwives who faced

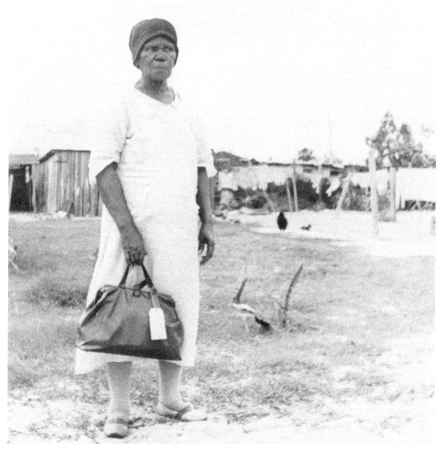

Figure 4.1. An African American midwife makes a visit in Broward County, ca. 1933. Courtesy of the State Library of Florida.

problems in their practices. And finally, in this case, it was an example of a midwife rejecting one of an extensive list of old superstitions and panaceas used by many of her white and African American counterparts.

On another level, the photograph and accompanying note reflect Graves's rapport with the midwives and her degree of empathy in a shared goal—quite simply to save mothers' and infants' lives. Graves's ability to communicate with the midwives, to root out the dangerous ones and even the incompetent ones, and teach the more able ones the safer methods of delivery stands in contrast to the general wave of public health nurses who, as Molly Ladd-Taylor has pointed out, stereotyped midwives for their ignorance and aligned it with lack of intelligence.[3] Laurie Jean Reid revealed that she "loathed the midwife."[4] In contrast, Graves understood their world. "It is hard for us old ones cause we got to disremember and l'arn all these new fangled ways of ketchin' babies," Graves recalled one midwife lamenting. And to be clear, Graves added that this midwife "was not being impertinent, but merely stating a fact."[5]

Whether working during or after the Sheppard-Towner Act program, Graves's task was to implement federal and/or state policies at a grassroots level. Yet many of her methods were not taught by nursing schools, the Children's Bureau, or any public health course. She evolved special ways to advance the maternal and infant welfare program and carry the message of healthy living and safe deliveries to rural women. She stood out among the state health nurses for the way she became the bridge to bring medical reforms to the midwives and rural women in the underserved communities. She drew others to her cause, colleagues and the next generation of state health nurses, touching them with her stories and inspiring them with an optimistic outlook. The African American Ethel J. Kirkland (1910–1985) joined the team in 1934 and summed up Graves as a "very sweet and devout Christian woman" but with fire in her actions. She added "the problems of sanitation and proper care were tackled with religious fever, which may not have been in the book, but after all Jule Graves was the book."[6]

In 1930, when the new graduate Lalla Mary Goggans (1906–1987) arrived at the State Board of Health, it was Graves and Joyce Ely who assisted her practically by showing her how to develop ways to interact with rural women and midwives. After her tenure in Perry, Ely had joined Graves at the State Board of Health in 1928. "I was truly amazed at their ability to speak the language of the midwives," Goggans said of Graves and Ely. "This I finally learned to do, but it took time." Kirkland noted that Graves's drive to serve Florida's mothers and infants took her along "some mighty dark and devious paths" to yield results. Kirkland added that she felt particularly qualified to comment on Graves's work because she followed her along those paths. She observed Graves firsthand to see her work among mothers and midwives as well as her lasting influence among public health nurses of the state. "Miss Julie was utterly color-blind. I

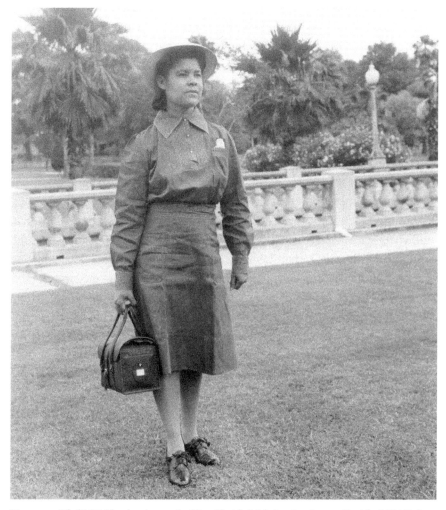

Figure 4.2. Ethel J. Kirkland arrives at the West Florida Midwives Institute at Florida A&M College in Tallahassee, 1933. Courtesy of the State Library of Florida.

never knew her to indicate that she knew whether a person was black or white," concluded Kirkland.[7]

In a state defined by its Jim Crow laws and culture, Kirkland's comment that Graves was colorblind requires context. Graves's drive nourished the overall public health mission to address maternal and infant deaths and maiming due to improper delivery procedures that profoundly affected the black and white people of Florida who were living out of the reach of well-trained doctors. The task that began with the Sheppard-Towner Act program and carried through to the civil rights movement necessitated that the state health nurses continue a rigorous program of finding cases, teaching health principles, and supervising midwives throughout the state. As Reid pointed out, midwives were an easier target to educate than physicians were, a point confirmed in a report from a White House conference in 1930 indicating that the responsibility for physician education lay with medical schools: "The ultimate problem of good obstetrics lies first in medical schools turning out men who are well trained in the fundamental principles and practice of obstetrics." The report recommended that all babies be delivered by obstetricians or doctors trained in obstetrics. The reality facing Florida's State Board of Health, however, was that there were too few doctors to serve Florida's large and diverse population. Furthermore, Florida was one of the states that fit into the White House conference committee's acknowledgment that "midwives are still needed in certain rural localities because of racial and economic conditions."[8] That the black and rural poor had no alternative but to engage midwives for deliveries was aptly illustrated by one new doctor who arrived in Ocala to start his practice in 1939. He found the "good paying people were jealously guarded and protected from all new practitioners" by the established doctors living in the area. He was left to glean his living from "unsuspected tourists."[9]

In the 1930s few black and rural folk could embrace the mainstream cultural trend toward hospital births that favored the male obstetrician over the midwife. Grace Higgs, the Miami-based public health nurse and supervisor of midwives, argued that it was simply not by choice that black women were dependent on midwives. Unless they had an emergency, Higgs noted, their race excluded them from admission for a normal delivery in Miami's segregated, publicly supported municipal Jackson Memorial Hospital.[10] One black doctor pointed out that if admitted in an emergency, a black woman could only look forward to treatment in the "dilapidated, unclean and generally undesirable area of the hospital."[11] Jackson Memorial Hospital was not an exception; in Florida most generally and throughout the South, racism, segregation, and economic factors were paramount to the black woman's use of a midwife. As Jackson was unavailable, the private African American Christian Hospital was open to those who could afford to pay.

But adding another layer of complexity, several black registered nurses noted that for most black women of Bahamian heritage during the Jim Crow era in Dade County, engaging a midwife was a part of their own cultural practice with major practical advantages. A midwife stayed, "no matter how many hours labor took, she didn't leave." She was there to supervise other children and sometimes provide food too. Verneka Silva remembered that her grandmother Ellen Stirrup, a midwife, "rode a bicycle. In the basket she would have the hot water and black bag and also food because she would always carry something for the mother to eat because at times there was no food in the home."[12] Yet for black or poor white women, having no choice but to engage a midwife formed an underlying layer to the fabric of society that Graves and her counterparts were powerless to change. If their goal was to save lives, the challenge was to find ways to work around the cultural mores of the state.

Notwithstanding the tension surrounding the racial fears created by Jim Crow customs, Graves soldiered on in her own manner almost defying custom at times. Her own words seem to clarify Kirkland's point that her manner was colorblind. On one occasion Graves jotted in her notes that she arrived in "a bad part of town . . . undid coat collar so white collar on uniform could show and walked back to where a col. man was. Asked him to tell me where a certain house was." Verbal and visual identification made people immediately aware of Graves's profession and task. When she met strangers she immediately identified herself as a "state nurse." The man not only obliged but offered to escort her. Graves accepted his offer with kind words. "You don't know how glad I'll be," she said.[13] Graves utilized her nurse's uniform to smooth the way, but she also offered an insight into how she reached in every direction to seek help from people, both white and black.

From the African American man's point of view, his willingness to escort Graves could have placed him in danger. Jennifer Ritterhouse has pointed out that African American men were often cautious about exposing themselves to any lone contact with white women lest they were accused of sexual assault, a pretext for lynching and Jim Crow laws alike. The fear of violence was perhaps more likely at the forefront of the African American man's consciousness than Graves's. Moreover, from the perspective of many white southerners, the color line was reinforced not only with the threat of violence but also a racial etiquette that preserved the custom that blacks were inferior and should be deferential to whites. The exchange between Graves and the man who helped her find an address spoke to the way two strangers put their faith in each other. Graves revealed her uniform to initiate the meeting, offering a way to ease tension. The incident also seems to illustrate Graves's lack of commitment to the customary racial etiquette, as Ritterhouse has noted, that blacks were not supposed to be treated "with the same respect and politeness that whites demanded for themselves."[14] While Kirkland's statement that Graves "never knew whether a person was black or white" could not have literally been true, she suggested that Graves had a more open mind to race relations. Such an attitude would have a profound effect on collaboration with community members as well as among her professional colleagues.

Jule O. Graves, "the Book"

"Miss Julie was a gentle, soft spoken seemingly naïve Southern maiden lady," remembered the future health office Dr. Wilson Sowder when he arrived in Florida in 1940.[15] Graves was born in St. Johns County in 1881 and spent her childhood in Florida. Her parents, the land developer and farmer Albert Graves and Mary Rose (Sue) Floyd hailed from Savannah, Georgia. "My dear little daughter does so much to help me," wrote Mary Rose to her sister when Jule was ten. Farm life in Florida, the cooking, washing, sewing, tending the crops, feeding the chickens, and coping with frosts on the orange groves was a life in contrast to Mary Rose's early life before the war living on Belleview Plantation in Camden County, Georgia. "Poverty is not calculated to brighten one," she lamented, offering an insight into Jule's formative years. While enduring practical hardships, Mary Rose took up her prolific pen to write short stories, often seeped in her memories of life at Belleview. She used the vernacular to bring her characters to life, a skill she handed down to Jule.[16]

Jule's motivation to begin a nursing career at Savannah's Park View Sanitarium in 1911 is unclear. The burgeoning nursing profession had gained force in the South, but a nursing career was still an exceptional decision for white, southern, literate women of this era. Perhaps her motivation was the poverty of her youth or a void in her life after the death of her mother in 1901 or something larger revolving around the world's work, a goal in common with many new women of the New South. She had all the attributes of a "new woman" that were captured in a 1917 toast to the twentieth-century women of North Carolina: "progressive but not bold; active and vigorous, but not pushing; independent and self sufficient, but not mannish, with sweetness of manner, gentleness of spirit and a growing desire to take part in the world's work."[17] For Graves, her world's work played out in Florida. After a summer course at Peabody College in Nashville in 1926, she arrived at the State Board of Health in Florida just in time for the hurricane and to begin, Ethel Kirkland noted, "giving her life to changing" the status quo of Florida's midwifery situation.[18]

Graves was not unlike many southern women who turned their gender prescriptions to their advantage and utilized soft-spoken language in pursuing goals of working for the public good.[19] As her writings reflect, Graves elicited reforms by layering her professional status with charisma, one of the key ingredients of southern ladyhood. Her charming ways helped her track down many midwives in rural north Florida, jotting notes as she saw firsthand the consequences of their work. "Uncle Ab," for example, was one of the male midwives she encountered who demonstrated the conditions that some Florida mothers and infants faced and the dire need for midwifery reform. She wrote a note on the back of a photograph describing Uncle Ab's deliveries: "Has delivered his last wife of most of their 14 children. His last wife 'went in' October '32, and died one month after delivery. Baby died at 6 weeks. This 72 year old colored man was called in to deliver a white woman latter part of '32. An internal examination was made. Baby died supposedly of tetanus on the 8th day."[20]

Often midwives' lives and work were intertwined with folk practices that had dangerous results. In one example, she found that a midwife had placed a makeshift pessary into a woman's vagina made from a fried egg inserted into an empty tobacco bag. The woman was left with the "shaking chills some days later." In another instance, a white woman was taken to hospital with pain in the lower abdomen, where the attending physician discovered a mass in the vagina resembling "oakum, soft strings or ravelings."[21] Graves listed traditions and often harmful ways country folk embraced as the only means they knew to kill pain, ward off diseases, and cure illness:

For excessive nausea secure a black chicken, must not have a single light colored feather, and steep slowly on the back of a stove. Undrawn and unpicked.

To insure an easy quick delivery, set her old man's hat on her head.

To cure after pains put a sharp plow share, knife or scissors under mother's bed to "cut the pains."

To cure sore eyes in the new born infant put milk [in the eyes] from the mother's breast.

To keep a husband, or lover constant put a little of the menstrual exchange in his drink.

To stop fits or convulsions, one live wood louse every other day until either seven or nine have been swallowed. To be most efficacious they should be swallowed head first and alive.[22]

To further illustrate the gravity of harmful "cures," Graves wrote one of her "Florida stories" about an encounter with conjuring and embellished the incident with dialect and conversation. In a visit to a remote area, Graves asked a country woman to identify the midwives of the area, using the folk phrase "catching babies." She identified herself as a state health nurse who taught midwives the best methods to deliver babies and help them with some births. The country woman then related to Graves that she knew of a woman "very sick with fits." In rural Florida during this era, often African Americans linked their medical folklore beliefs to consultation with the voodoo priest or priestess who had the power to cast spells, whether for good or evil.[23] Knowing the prevalence of such "conjurers" in the area, Graves asked whether the sick woman fell and bit her lip. She also asked "who conjured her." The woman said, "Thank God you know an' please go see her now." Based on Graves's response, the woman assumed Graves to be knowledgeable about country ways. It evidently made her more trustworthy to the woman. The woman directed Graves to the sick woman, and Graves noted that she treated her for the dangerous hypertensive disorder that could lead to convulsions. Graves concluded, "I supposed the sick woman had eclampsia and guessed about the 'kunjer' part."[24] It is unclear how Graves treated the woman. Severe preeclampsia could produce cerebral and visual disturbances and would have been dangerous for that "conjured" pregnant women as well as the unborn infant. Graves's only recourse in the field was most likely to facilitate a conservative treatment that involved bed rest, sedation, and careful monitoring.[25]

The episode highlights a method Graves employed to seek out midwives and indicates the importance of having an intimate understanding of the cultural and religious tenets of the communities. Graves found conjuring to be a "real menace to the colored mothers and babies; a contributory cause for the high maternal and infant death rate."[26] She was not sympathetic, exactly, but met people where they were to not only stress prevention of disease but treatment as well. Addressing communities steeped in folklore required an intense collaboration with the midwives. Many of the midwives proved competent and trustworthy and helped the nurses find those who were not. African American church ministers also supported the nurses' and midwives' move to root out harmful conjuring practices. They reproached church members who conferred with conjure priests.[27]

Graves's intimate connection with country folk also shows in her ability to win over people through storytelling. By drawing upon the regional love for tall tales, she persuaded people who were not immediately responsive to her "high falutin notions." On one occasion Graves had run out of silver nitrate drops necessary to put into babies' eyes after delivery to prevent neonatal ophthalmia.[28] As the nearest drugstore was several miles away, she needed someone to obtain the medication while she remained with the mother. Intuition told her a tall tale would serve her purpose. Earlier she had spotted a sorrel mare nearby and requested that one of the men ride that particular horse to obtain medicine from the drugstore. She wrote, "The fact that a sorrel mare had to be ridden to make the medicine effective was something the poor fellow could not understand." The man willingly galloped off to town on the horse to fulfill Graves's request.[29] While some might argue that Graves's tale fooled people into accepting the dominance of her class and culture, others might recognize her attempt to save an infant's eyesight as justification to entice people to accept the benefits that modern health care could bring. The underlying message of the story is that Graves became a bridge to modern medical care for a population that often relied only on folk medicine or divine healing. Although devious and manipulative, Graves's use of indirect persuasion was for her a means to the end.

Graves must have repeated her story to Kirkland and others, reflecting the long tradition of southern storytelling when people told stories on their way home from church or on their way to market or gathered at the fireside in the evening.[30] As demonstrated in Kirkland's repetition of Graves's stories, the southern mode of storytelling often included jokes about naiveté to arouse laughter.[31] Perhaps the people knew it was a yarn that helped them to smooth the way to accepting Graves's demand. Importantly, the story became one that obtained an immediate favorable response to saving a baby's sight as well as one Graves could tell other nurses to help them develop more fluid relations with rural people.

Graves drew on this gift for creative storytelling as a tactic to engage people and help her build bridges to reach rural women. When the storytelling technique worked well, she repeated the narrative to reach more women and men, too. One story showed how she circumvented a woman's religious beliefs to treat her children for hookworm.[32] When driving along a country road, Graves noticed six children showing signs of hookworm disease. Hookworm infestation was heaviest among rural children where sanitary conditions in homes and schools were poor and children became infected and reinfected with the parasite larvae by walking barefoot on contaminated ground. Likely the children were without shoes with visible signs as described by one doctor as "very pale & anaemic & has other symptoms common to the complaint, enervated, & showing some bloat."[33] Graves wrote, "I told them if they would get in the car I would take them home."[34] The children got a lift, and more importantly Graves found a way to seek out their mother.

At first the mother's response was negative to Graves's offer of treatment. Many rural people of Florida, including this mother, embraced the Pentecostal theology of the Church of God. Church of God followers believed in divine healing and viewed physicians and modern medicine with suspicion. The mother replied that "her religion forbade the use of doctors or medicines."[35] Though respectful of her beliefs, Graves happened to remember that the religion of the Church of God considered the body to be the temple of the Holy Ghost, and she recognized the significance the church's doctrine would have on her work. She effectively maneuvered her health teaching around the church rules and into a concept this mother would accept. Graves made the connection for the woman by using an analogy of ridding vegetable plants of worms to keep the plants healthy. She asked the mother why she would not want to keep a child's body, "the Temple of the Holy Ghost," as clear of worms as a vegetable plant. "I hadn't thought about that," the mother replied. The woman assured Graves that if she left the specimen bottles "she would fix 'em up," and if the specimens came back from the laboratory positive, she said, "I'll give 'em the medicine." Graves was so pleased with the effectiveness of her explanation that she later used it on the "school board man also a member of the Church of God."[36] By knowing and understanding the culture of the people she wished to serve, Graves took quiet action to negotiate around the obstacles, in contrast to Laurie Jean Reid's vocal rage about religious fatalism.

Graves's Footsteps and Lalla Mary Goggans

When Jule Graves became a state health nurse for Florida in 1926, Lalla Mary Goggans was embarking on her own nursing career at the Orange School of Nursing in Orlando and gained experience at De Lee's Lying-In Hospital in Chicago. After that training, Goggans had a unique opportunity to develop her career in public health as one of Laurie Jean Reid's protégés and one of Graves's mentees. Reid arranged for her to attend postgraduate training in public health in Virginia, sponsored by the Florida Federation of Women's Clubs. Goggans completed the course at the College of William and Mary in Richmond, Virginia, in June 1930, after the Sheppard-Towner Act program expired and Reid retired. Armed with her formal public health training, Goggans became one of Florida's state health nurses representing a new generation of budding leaders of public health nursing for the state and later for the nation.[37]

One of the first lessons Goggans learned in those first months was the literal route to conduct her path of reform—an introduction to the perils of driving in a harsh environment and an obstacle Graves knew too well. In June 1930 floodwater from the swollen Caloosahatchee River stranded the townspeople of La Belle in Hendry County. "I received word from the people in La Belle about the Caloosahatchee flood." Graves wrote in her notes. "They wanted me to come at once re prenatal cases. The Woman's Clubs at Fort Myers had given me layettes." Graves attempted to deliver the prenatal supplies to the marooned women, but her car got stuck in the floodwater. "I went slowly, there was already a little water in the car. Then the car lurched," Graves wrote. "I knew I couldn't get out of that place." Rescued but undeterred, the following day she simply "put on dungarees and waded out." When the water was too deep, she borrowed a rowboat to get through.[38] Such determination fired Goggans's ambition.

Graves led by example. An underlying message that Goggans soon grasped was that difficult travel was not a deterrent to reach a favorable outcome. Driving in the Everglades was a unique Florida challenge. After inspecting the eyes

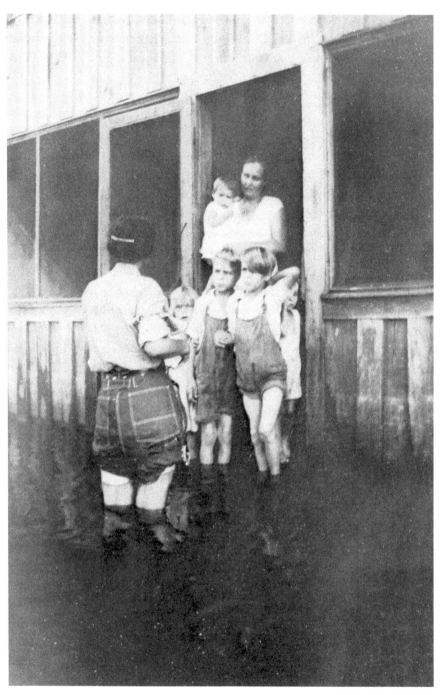

Figure 4.3. During the La Belle floods of June 1930, Jule Graves delivers a layette donated by the Fort Myers Woman's Club. Courtesy of the State Library of Florida.

of schoolchildren, Graves wanted to visit with the parents of one little girl whose eyesight was dangerously poor. The teacher advised against the move because "her father is a bootlegger and the road is long and bad and I certainly wouldn't go." Graves did not heed her advice but ultimately found that the teacher had not underestimated the driving difficulties. By the time Graves reached the house she was in "a typical swamp." The father, however, was receptive to Graves's recommendations and later followed through with taking the girl to a visit to an eye specialist. Graves felt amply repaid for the terrible journey that even got worse on her return home when she was forced to negotiate a floating bridge. "It was a scary looking place and bridge," she recalled, "and when the bridge began to go down, one of the biggest water moccasins I ever saw wiggled out."[39]

Graves's difficult travels that took her into the Everglades also drew out the significance of Florida's distinctive environment to the Seminoles who found sanctuary amid the swamps after the nineteenth-century Seminole Wars. After World War I, clubwomen on the east and west coasts of Florida had taken a great interest in the welfare of the Seminoles by publicizing their living conditions and securing medicines and the services of a doctor.[40] The year Graves arrived at the State Board of Health, in 1926, Julia Hanson, the federation's chair of the Division of Seminole Indians, facilitated her introduction to the tribe living near the Tamiami Trail. In her role as the State Board of Health's intermediary, Graves facilitated health intercessions to the Seminole families by linking with the clubwomen as well as the philanthropic Seminole Indians Association of Florida directed by W. Stanley Hanson, Julia's husband.[41] By the time Charlotte Conrad, the first US Public Health Service nurse, arrived at the reservation in 1934 to deliver federally backed interventions, Graves had laid the groundwork to develop those relations.[42]

Goggans would not miss that Graves did not fit into the pattern of other public health nurses who visited Native Americans in other parts of the country. According to Molly Ladd-Taylor, most were critical of customs and practices such as children's diets or babies' tight clothing.[43] There is no indication Graves was shocked by Seminole child-rearing customs. Rather, her photographs replete with her own notes speak to her connection and bond with them. Her caption on the back of one photograph indicates that the Cypress couple named their daughter, born on May 23, 1933, Julia Graves Cypress.[44] The development of such intimacy between the Cypress family and Graves would have taken time. According to an observer who accompanied Graves

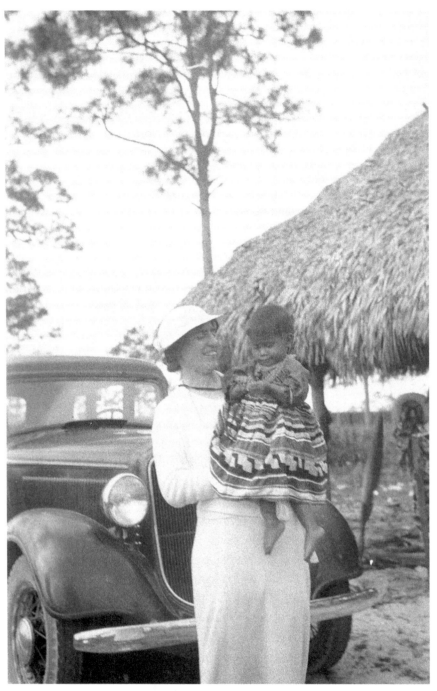

Figure 4.4. Jule Graves holds Julia Graves Cypress at a temporary camp in Immokalee, ca. 1933. Courtesy of the State Library of Florida.

on a visit, "The Indians loved her; even the men who were usually so reserved smiled at her."[45] Again, to elicit such a response from the Indians required repeated visits. Graves encouraged Joyce Ely and Lalla Goggans to join her on some occasions. Inspired by Graves's lead, they too became members of the Seminole Indian Association and helped clear the path for Conrad to follow.[46]

After a few months of working alongside Graves, Ely, and other state health nurses, Goggans set out to tackle the many health care needs made worse by the Depression in ten rural counties of the Florida Panhandle. She noted that the counties of westernmost Florida were the poorest in the state, marked by "poverty, hunger, deprivation, lack of health care of any kind, [and] few physicians (some of the counties had none)."[47] Goggans was born in Live Oak in Suwannee County and found her knowledge of the geographical and cultural environment essential in her move to care for mothers and children, but even that was not enough. She credited the success of her work not to her formal public health training but to the mentoring she received from the older Sheppard-Towner nurses.[48]

Learning to drive a Model A Ford came first, but heading into rural communities caused Goggans great difficulty in negotiating the sand roads or no roads and streams with few sound bridges. She recalled that when driving over the rickety bridges she "fell through three times" before she learned to "stay on the good planks." Following in Graves's footsteps, she also waded creeks or hopped over barbed-wire fences and proceeded alone to isolated areas to make personal contact with the midwives. "I conducted classes for midwives in Negro churches which were often located in the tall uncut woods; in county Court Houses, or wherever I could find a place to meet," she wrote.[49] Goggans's recollections of her journeys and the rural settings for the midwives' instruction shine a light on Florida's geography and landscape composition but seemingly ignore the underlying prevailing racial tension and possible dangers for a white woman to travel alone.

The meetings with the midwives brought the races together in a shared goal to deliver better care for mothers and infants. The midwives club meetings were important ways to develop mutual understanding between the state health nurses and the midwives. In the South, the friendly group meetings took on an aura of a church service to respect the midwives' religious beliefs.[50] One Florida midwife revealed, "I shore did have to pray. 'Cause when I do go on cases, you know, I want the Lord to go with me where I could have success. I'd asked him."[51] Many midwives believed their work was

a calling from God. Another midwife said, "I was called from God, and I delivered 'em all. . . . God gave me the job."[52] Typically the nurses leveraged the
concept of the calling with a prayer and a hymn sung by all when conducting classes about cleanliness, personal hygiene, and birth reporting. Yet the
liking of the religious aspect of the meetings was not always one-sided, and
a more fluid relation between the parties sometimes occurred than scholars have acknowledged. Goggans was clear that she enjoyed that part of the
meeting as well. The hymn "Climbing Jacob's Ladder" was her favorite, and
she was moved with the midwives' rendition of a special prayer to keep her
in good stead: "Lord keep your hand on the steering wheel of our nurse and
steer her right for she is so young." There was mutual warmth; the midwives
referred to Goggans as "our nurse," and Goggans referred to the midwives as
"my midwives."[53] From Goggans's perspective the classes were "joyous occasions" for all participants. And from the midwives' perspective, one midwife
concluded, "us loves our meetings."[54]

Goggans related the way she worked through the many layers of cultural
and professional differences to enlist the midwives as allies to improve the
health care of women. Most generally midwives welcomed the opportunity
to help save lives. They enjoyed the social companionship with others and
liked the recognition for their work and suggestions to facilitate it.[55] "We
tried to do the right thing," one midwife recalled when recounting her work
in the 1930s. "As soon as that baby's born, I got to call the health department.
But they never did find anything wrong."[56] Goggans imparted the standard
instructions: no interference with the natural process of labor in any way,
the importance of cleanliness, and the necessity of seeking a physician's aid
for any complications. "I inspected their bags and gave demonstrations on
hand washing, perineal care and care of mother's nursing nipples," she noted.
Yet from Goggans's perspective, the midwives taught her as well as learned
from her. "If I faltered in any way it was the midwives who held me up on
every learning side," she wrote.[57] Perhaps the midwives felt that Goggans had
faltered by not finding all the midwives in her area and therefore missed the
opportunity to save infants' eyesight and perhaps lives too, a tragedy that
prompted them to take action.

Taught by Graves to find innovative ways to relate to midwives and seek
their support, Goggans came up with a small demonstration to address the
high maternal death rate in one county. She collected beans in a jar, with each
bean representing one death. Evidently, several midwives did not want Gog-

gans to falter in her work and took her aside to report that many of the beans belonged to Aunt Becky. The information sent Goggans into the field to find Aunt Becky and investigate the reason for the deaths. She discovered that the only physician in that part of the county had taught Aunt Becky "new fangled ways" to do vaginal examinations and administer quinine and castor oil to begin labor.[58] All midwives were expected to call a physician for support if necessary, but this physician had shown how he was negligent in his practice to teach a midwife some techniques that placed women's and infants' lives at risk. He likely fell into what Mary Breckinridge of the Frontier Nursing Service in Kentucky dubbed "pseudo-doctors," practicing without the benefit of formal training.[59] Goggans was aware that by the mid-1920s, leaders in the field of obstetrics like Dr. Joseph De Lee, her mentor at the training school in Chicago, were gradually acknowledging doctors' part in the cause of high maternal mortality and calling for reforms.[60] But just as a professional blindfold strapped Terry and Reid, Goggans sidestepped the doctor's negligence. She had no other recourse but to inform the doctor that the State Board of Health had a policy concerning deliveries conducted by midwives that included forbidding midwives to do vaginal examinations. She evidently followed up later to make sure the midwife changed her practice, concluding that "she was not one of the best midwives, but was the only one in a very isolated section of the country."[61]

From Problem to Program

The uneasy relations between doctors and nurses played out within State Board of Health at a different level. Dr. Lucile Spire Blachly, a pediatrician from Oklahoma, became the director of the Florida Bureau of Child Hygiene and Public Health Nursing upon Reid's departure in January 1930. Immediately, Blachly implemented a child hygiene program similar to one that was working well in her home state of Oklahoma. Like Reid, she embraced a reform attitude no matter the consequences to the midwives' lives. Like Reid, her attitude toward public health reflected her endorsement of eugenic philosophy. In *Florida Health Notes* she made it clear that she intended to direct policy toward "the betterment of all children—therefore the race. Race betterment must come if our civilization is to survive."[62] While there is no question the state health nurses understood the imperative of reforming child health care, modernizing midwives' practices, excluding male midwives, and removing those midwives who could not be made competent, they employed innovative and kindly ways to become a bridge to modern health care. By attempting to institute reforms without seeking guidance from the state health nurses, Blachly placed a wedge in the relations between the nurses and the midwives, creating a tension over official policy.

Blachly welcomed the opportunity to push for reform ideals in Florida. She was keen to work with Dr. Henry Hanson, the state health officer, whom she admired for his accomplishments in public health.[63] Hanson had begun serving as Florida's state health officer in 1929 and believed, after Reid left, that a pediatrician could best serve as the director of the Bureau of Child Hygiene and Public Health Nursing. Evidently, Hanson had given little thought to the impact of assigning the directorship of public health nursing to a physician rather than a nurse and one who did not obtain advice from the experienced state health nurses who worked in the field and understood the way of life in rural areas. While the doctors and state health nurses shared goals to improve child health, Hanson's report indicates that Blachly ignored input from the state health nurses on how best to approach the reform of midwives. Hanson revealed that from the beginning of Blachly's employment, philosophical differences in outlook marred her relations with the state health nurses. By January 1932, the consequences of the discord came to a head. Hanson reported "an unfortunate incompatibility between the director and some of the older nurses developed which made it desirable to temporarily suspend the bureau for reorganization."[64]

From the start, Blachly marked her difference of opinion with the state health nurses by placing those midwives, "even though they were capable and conscientious to begin with," in the same category as some she acknowledged might be "few in number, who, ignorantly or purposely, are resorting to practices not approved."[65] Blachly intended to inaugurate a new state program that shared the state nurses' supervision of midwives with local health authorities having public health personnel.[66] As a first step, she requested that state health nurses conduct a "fact-finding" survey to assess the number of midwives in the state along with the midwives' personal information to include each one's name, address, age, length of service, education, number of deliveries, who had taught them, and the reason she became a midwife.[67] Many midwives conscientiously participated in the surveys and fulfilled another of Blachly's requirements, to help locate crippled children. Some midwives had delivered the children. The surveys could not have been completed without the midwives' collaboration. Hanson and Blachly reported, "There were 1,303 persons who delivered one or more babies in Florida in 1930 . . . [and] of this number 998 were 'licensed' midwives, 149 unlicensed midwives and 156 attendants other than midwives."[68] Blachly's announcement that "present instruction and supervision was inadequate" was not a point of contention with the state health nurses if she was referring to the number of state health nurses to cover the state.[69] Rather, their objection was to the way Blachly intended to implement changes.

Graves and her counterparts understood that even though many of the midwives were capable and conscientious, they were set in their ways and challenged by the task of reeducation. Blachly, on the other hand, decided on ways to improve the service delivery that was difficult for the midwives to understand. Graves recognized their problems. Her manner of teaching stood in stark contrast to Blachly's ideas of imposing midwifery reforms. The rapport between Florida's state health nurses and midwives was severely tested when Blachly implemented changes to the methods of delivery without affording the state health nurses time to explain the changes to midwives.[70]

Blachly determined that midwives had to "be kept abreast of the times." She decided that one of the best ways to improve service delivery was to revise Reid's "obsolete" *Manual for Midwives* and send a letter of instruction to midwives advising them of changes in procedure.[71] Blachly wanted the midwives to establish a sterile field when delivering babies and thus ordered them to buy razors to shave their patients prior to delivery and masks to cover their own noses and mouths, caps for their heads, and long white gowns to wear for the deliveries. According to Goggans, the older nurses responded with "fury" that the doctor had not consulted them before sending this letter to the midwives. They "were wild when they heard about the letter. It was a real blessing that not many of the granny midwives could read or write because they would not have understood this great change," she wrote.[72] By communicating directly with the midwives, Blachly ignored how the state health nurses were bridges between the board and the midwives.

The state health nurses had to hustle to the field to explain Blachly's changes and teach them why this "new 'fangled' equipment" was important. Blachly overlooked that many of the midwives were illiterate and found it difficult to "l'arn all these new fangled ways of ketchin' babies." She had not examined their perspective. Evidently, neither did she carefully consider how the letter did not make sense when terms of Florida's new midwifery law that was in draft included a provision for midwives who could not read the "*Manual for Midwives* intelligently and fill out the birth certificates legibly."[73] Those who were illiterate could seek a waiver by the health officer. Goggans herself had helped to draft the bill that became law in 1931.[74] Those who could read or otherwise somehow learned about the contents of the letter were puzzled. Some midwives were mystified at the thought of the razors. According to Goggans, they arrived at the meetings with "straight razors, shaving mugs and worn out shaving brushes."[75] The concept of shaving a patient was completely new to most midwives, and many did not want to comply with the instructions. Although practicing a few years later, one midwife explained her disdain for shaving women: "so many of 'em [women] I didn't shave. If they didn't want it, I didn't shave 'em. 'Cause I never was shaved for any of *my* children."[76]

In their position as intermediaries between the board and the midwives, the state health nurses found ways to help the midwives comply with Blachly's immediate demands. The confusion about the razors was cleared up when the nurses bought safety razors and resold them to midwives at cost. The masks, too, were perplexing to the midwives. Graves snapped a photograph of a midwife wearing one and trying to adhere to the misconceived directions. In a caption on the back she wrote that it was "her interpretation of nose and mouth mask . . . a cross between a tea strainer and a chloroform mask."[77] To help midwives comply with the new regulations, public health nurses prepared patterns for the caps, masks, and gowns so that midwives could make their own equipment. Yet there were further problems associated with the gowns that perhaps could have been avoided if the state health nurses had been afforded time to prepare the midwives adequately. A midwife had donned her gown without explaining the procedure to a mother in labor. "One midwife reported that when she came in to deliver the mother after a hand scrub, 'she took one look at me and hollered Klan! Klan! and took off running out the door.'"[78] The anguish caused to this mother could only have made the state health nurses even wilder by the orders being delivered without a true understanding of local situations. Blachly raised the state health nurses' ire when she took away their roles of intermediaries, leading to rounds of misunderstandings and in this case between the midwife and the frightened mother.

At the height of the Great Depression, Blachly's insistence upon rules that the midwives purchase razors and other equipment out of their own pockets intimates a blindness on her part to the economic realities of the population she was in charge of serving. Conversely, Goggans noted her personal anguish when her family members lost all their assets, but even this hardship paled in comparison to people's dire straits in west Florida, leaving her with images that haunted her for the rest of her life. Then, on January 15, 1932, a lack of funding compounded the inner discord in the department and forced the board to close the department's doors except for a skeleton staff. Only Joyce Ely and two other nurses remained.[79] Jule Graves left the state temporarily, Goggans returned to Orlando to try to find work as a private-duty nurse for a few months, and Blachly left Florida permanently.

Hanson reorganized the board so that the state health nurses were under the direction of a supervisory nurse who was familiar with the challenges facing public health nurses.[80] The move established a separate Division of Public Health Nursing. Later in the year, when the state health nurses trickled back, this small division consisted of only five state health nurses; two of them were Goggans and Graves, returning in August and September, respectively.[81] Joyce Ely became the state supervisor of midwives and acting chief nurse. Hanson would appoint a permanent director of public health nursing, Ruth Mettinger, in 1934 and with backing from the Federal Emergency Relief Administration funds, he promised "the development of an elaborate nursing program."[82]

Meanwhile, Goggans's position at the board afforded her greater authority when she returned for service in August 1932, a month prior to Graves's return. Goggans replaced Joyce Ely, who was awarded a Rockefeller fellowship to attend the first class for nurse-midwifery at the Maternity Center Association, Lobenstein Clinic, in New York and would be absent for ten months.[83] In fact, Ely's further education marked Florida as one of the few states with a nurse-midwife supervising the midwife program. During Ely's absence, Goggans had the credentials to take charge of the state program from the Jacksonville headquarters, but at the same time she remained responsible for the supervision of midwives in west Florida.

It was the midwives of west Florida who sparked Goggans's further role in strengthening the midwifery program. When her state responsibilities kept her in Jacksonville and prevented her from making all her rural visits, the midwives missed her and contacted Hanson to ask why she had not visited them.[84] In response, Goggans decided the best way to reach many midwives at one time was to implement a recommendation from the White House conference "to establish institutions in the South for the proper training of midwives." These institutes "would be a community responsibility."[85] Initiating the founding of the midwifery institutes where midwives could assemble for extensive learning experiences indicated how Goggans met the challenge to meet all the midwives in a timely manner from all her counties. Goggans enlisted the cooperation of Dr. J. R. Lee, president of A&M College in Tallahassee, and arranged the first Florida Midwife Institute to be held at the college from August 20 to 27, 1933. Each midwife was asked to pay one dollar for the week's room and board. Even though the Depression was upon them, 265 midwives paid the fee for the week's room and board to attend. The enthusiastic support from the community included clubwomen, who provided transportation where needed, members of the American Medical Association, who assisted with instruction, and others, who offered financial help with the fee.[86] Her initiative to bring everyone together, community members, midwives, doctors, and nurses, is a prime example of Goggans's role as a bridge for health reform.

The key to the success of the institute, according to Goggans, was the community support and in particular the cooperation of the African American public health nurses Margaret Johnson from the Duval County Health Department and Irene Odell McGreen from the Leon County Health Department, who helped to organize the event.[87] Graves returned to her work in time to participate in the institute and like all the public health nurses was moved with emotion to hear the midwives lift their voices in song. The practice of midwifery had become more regulated, and the midwives now licensed were proud of their new status. They had become so accustomed to their regulation gowns that they wore them to class. "Wearing them was their idea," reported Goggans. Clearly, the midwives appreciated the instruction, as one conveyed in a letter to Hanson. The midwife wrote, "Dr. Hanson i just don't Express just how i thank you for haven we mid wifes such a teaching as we did get from so many presons and all Was so good I doe thank you for our Being her We leaving here With harts and mind full intention to Live up our teachen thank you."[88] The growing cooperation and mutual trust continued as many of the midwives helped to organize the next institute in Tampa later in year.[89] "I realize now how much these midwives taught me," concluded Goggans many years later, without reflecting on the impact of the social construction of health on them or on the lives of the women they served.[90]

Taking the Lead

By 1935 the midwife program was in full swing with the leadership smoothly transitioned from the nurse-midwife Joyce Ely to Jule Graves.[91] The midwifery program had begun to rely on local supervisors, black and white, to oversee the midwives in their communities and arrange the monthly classes and pre-natal clinics.[92] In 1933, of eighteen public health nurse supervisors, four were African American: Irene Odell McGreen for Leon County, Carrie Emanuel for Dade County, Zula Bonner for West Palm Beach City, and Rosa Brown for West Palm Beach County.[93] When 89 percent of the midwives were black, the appointments of black public health nurses as local supervisors represented a professional achievement that began to blur the boundaries of race in the supervision of Florida's midwifery program.[94] Rosa Brown offered insight by noting that the "direct supervision of 11 colored and two white midwives in our county was turned over to me by the State Board of Health."[95] The appoint-ments of Brown and her counterparts was a start at least to allow public health nurses to mirror the communities they served. The leadership recognized their value. Goggans pointed out that she did not consider her African American counterparts as her professional, moral, or social inferiors. Rather, she said, it was Johnson and McGreen who "encouraged her."[96]

Further quiet blurring of racial lines came in 1936 with the appointment of Ethel Kirkland as the State Midwife Teacher and an assistant to Graves. Her rise to this position at the State Board of Health began in 1934 when the Division of Public Health Nursing expanded and began a new era under the leadership of Ruth Mettinger. Mettinger's first assignment was to supervise the Florida Emergency Relief Administration nursing program, which "provided for 15 supervisors and 275 county nurses."[97] Kirkland and her sister Flossie Brown Lewes, recent graduates of St. Philips Hospital in Richmond, Virginia, were among the first nurses in the program. Just as Graves had taken Gog-gans under her wing, Goggans, the supervisor for west Florida, mentored the new graduates. All shared identical philosophies.[98] From the start Kirkland "wanted to do something about the disgracefully high mortality among the new mothers and the new born, and upgrade the practices of the thousands of amateur midwives."[99]

The midwifery program became specialized to save lives and improve mid-wives' practices; it was not incorporated into the general program but grew with the dynamic leaders to guide it. Graves's vibrant direction never failed to distinguish her as a powerful presence within the State Board of Health. In 1940, Marshall Doss, the director of the State Board of Health Bureau of Nar-cotics, introduced himself to the prospective state health officer, Dr. Wilson T. Sowder, as the "Director, Bureau of Narcotics and Chief Consultant to Miss Ju-

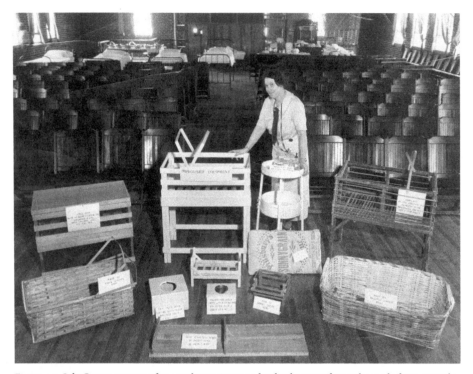

Figure 4.5. Jule Graves prepares for a midwives institute by displaying infant cribs made from everyday materials, ca. 1935. Graves engaged the WPA to make cribs to help women prepare for giving birth and prevent infant deaths by having infants sleep in their own bassinettes. Courtesy of the State Library of Florida.

lie Graves." One reason Doss gave himself such a title was a seemingly innocent request from Graves that he help her fix a problem with her sawed-off shotgun. Sowder recalled, "Mr. Doss was horrified and said, 'Miss Julie don't you know it's a federal offence to have a sawed off shotgun in your possession?'" Graves was dismissive of the law, explaining that it was merely to shoot rattlesnakes.[100] Kirkland repeated the story of the incident with a comment that Graves did indeed meet many rattlesnakes on her journeys. However, Kirkland's conclusion that one could only "imagine the chagrin of such a proper and decorous little lady finding herself a criminal" seems inconsistent with Graves's personality.[101] Certainly, environmental dangers stood out in Graves's notes. She was perfectly comfortable to brush them aside and content to carry the weapon to protect herself. But part of her story—and that of the state health nurses—is missing. Graves did not record any encounter with a hostile, menacing, or even nasty person. She led the program with an optimistic outlook. Her records speak to her goal, even if they suggest the undercurrent of danger facing the state health nurses generally as they traveled the state alone.

From 1935 through 1947, when she retired, the cheery Graves brought her creativity to the fore. At first, she engaged a Works Progress Administration arts and crafts class to fashion infant cribs from everyday supplies. This helped new mothers who struggled to find resources, prepare for the births of their babies, and prevent infant deaths by stressing the necessity that the infant sleep in his or her own improvised bassinette. She also designed two life-size dolls, one black and one white, with mechanical features to demonstrate childbirth and facilitate midwives in their learning. She particularly wanted "the fetus to look and feel like a normal baby." Again, she turned to the Works Progress Administration. She wrote, "They told me I could tell the men just what I wanted and they would be glad to help."[102] Graves used the life-size "Chase dolls," so named for their demonstration value, at club meetings. She often gleefully repeated the story that one time a "nosey individual" took a peep into the trunk and rushed off to the police of Fernandina Beach to report that Graves was carrying dead bodies in her car! During her tenure, the dolls, for which she eventually received a patent, had become real members of the board. On departing from a meeting, one midwife said, "Miz Chase, let me rench (wring) your hand, and come back and see us again soon."[103]

Creating a warm and friendly atmosphere continued to serve Graves well. Kirkland captured the midwives' receptiveness to Graves's teaching and their will to improve their practices. Some "walked 10 or 14 miles, others went hungry to attend the classes," and for her part, Graves was "never too tired to give extra time and effort" to them in turn.[104] Graves initiated a special ceremony when she encouraged many problem midwives to retire by giving them special recognition. This ceremony "removed the possibility of needlessly hurting the old midwife's feelings, as she feels that she is not simply discarded," Graves noted.[105] The midwives provided a vital service. For again, in the rural areas there was a dearth of alternatives.

First working alongside Graves and then assuming the leadership of the midwife program, Kirkland was credited by her peers as one of the most outstanding public health nurses in Florida and one who greatly strengthened the midwifery program. Armed with a master's degree in public health from the University of Michigan and like Ely and Graves among the earliest to become certified nurse midwives, Kirkland spent her forty-year career both in the field and rewriting the board's rules and regulations pertaining to the midwives' practices. They were, she remembered, "years of toil." The uphill climb during those years must have been compounded by Ethel Kirkland's personal struggle as an outsider within the State Board of Health. It is striking that whereas Jule Graves made her own book, if Kirkland was to successfully reach the community she wished to serve, she could absolutely make no waves. Kirkland was vocal about Jule Graves's influence, while insights into her own life and work depend on scant sources to piece together. Importantly, one exceptional source reveals the racial tensions and the hostility during the 1950s that targeted Kirkland and threatened to undermine her work (see chapter 5, pages 152–53).

If the link that ran between Graves, Goggans, and Kirkland promoted an optimistic outlook to improve people's lives, it was also one that fostered a quiet social activism within the board. It was a means that provided a firm footing to support a biracial female support system, not specifically to disturb the relations between the races but to work together as bridges between the board and Florida's diverse communities. The rapport they developed with the midwives was the key to their success in their work. Goggans reflected, "Jule had a great respect and love for the 'granny midwives,' and so did I!"[106] As Graves guided, supported, taught, and inspired her younger colleagues in the field, she imparted this quiet social activism to Goggans, who in turn conveyed it to her mentees. Goggans exemplified how her rapport with Kirkland and the county nurses McGreen and Johnson fostered the biracial relations between nursing colleagues. Although working in the face of racism was a fact of life for Kirkland, her white colleagues were supportive. When Kirkland called Graves "utterly color-blind," she was speaking in a context of Graves's work among rural women and midwives. However, there is a sense that she was also speaking from her own experience as an African American woman. It speaks to the beginnings of a real transformation in race relations in the nursing profession. Such a quiet social activism foreshadowed the rumblings toward the integration of the professional black and white nursing associations—with Florida leading the way.

5

Battling On without Fanfare for
Better Health Conditions, 1934 to 1964

"The uniform of a public health nurse is in itself a badge of courage," wrote Ruth Mettinger, the director of the Bureau of Public Health Nursing in the April 1943 edition of *Florida Health Notes*. She was responding to the public's criticism of many of Florida's public health nurses when they did not race into the US Army or Navy at the onset of the United States' involvement in World War II. After Pearl Harbor, 15,000 graduate nurses left health agencies, hospitals, and private-duty assignments to join the military. Mettinger, always aware that favorable public opinion strengthened the public health nursing service, made it clear to the critics that they "did not understand the great war service public health nurses are rendering right here at home"—and for Mettinger "home" meant Florida. Many rural areas of Florida had become centers of war industry and military concentration. The increased population added to the public health nurses' workload of seeking out Florida's poorly served residents. Even so, they "leave no vital battle station on the home front unmanned," wrote Mettinger. To enlighten the public further she continued that the nurses who stayed stateside were "doing their part towards winning the war just as surely as though they served on the more obvious battle front." She implied that the misunderstandings and questions were simply not fair. They could make a public health nurse "feel like a slacker. It sometimes takes a greater courage and loyalty to give service when there is no fanfare," she concluded.[1] These words guided her career in Florida from 1922 to 1963 and held a special resonance. During World War I she had faced a similar dilemma—would she join the Army Nurse Corps or remain in the public health field to serve without fanfare in Virginia?

Mettinger was just two years out of nursing school and engaged in public health work in Virginia when she responded to Jane Delano's call for active service in the Red Cross Nursing Service. Born and raised in Sanford, Florida, she had graduated from St. Timothy's Hospital Training School in Roxborough, Pennsylvania, the location of her parents' home before they moved south to Florida during the mid-1880s.[2] From her training school to her public health work in Pennsylvania and on to Virginia, Mettinger's personality and manner along with her nursing and teaching skills impressed her supervisors. It was no surprise, therefore, when her supervisor in Richmond in 1918 requested that the Red Cross issue her a "special chevron . . . to continue her present important work" in Virginia. Mettinger deferred her plan and mustered her own "greater courage," a mettle that served her throughout her tenure in Florida.[3] She was one of Florida's first Sheppard-Towner Act nurses in 1922; four years later, she continued to serve Floridians as the Red Cross state and regional field representative. In 1934 she secured her position as director of public health nursing for the State Board of Health to become the public health nurses' standard bearer. Her overall public health nursing experience along with her grasp of Florida's environmental and cultural challenges served her well to lead the vital members of the three-horse team for almost thirty years, a team that thrived best with the support of an educated citizenry.

County Health Units: Facilitating the Public Health Nurses' Reach

When Mettinger took up the reins of leadership in 1934, the state health officer Henry Hanson won a strong ally to plan and administer effective public health nursing programs that were particularly needed in the rural areas. "We must have [public health nurses] for the rural communities where doctors will not go," Hanson insisted.[4] Living conditions in rural Florida and the slum districts of cities continued to be of low standards, causing major health problems. Many of the poorer white and African American citizens disregarded or had limited access to proper sanitary conveniences, making them fertile grounds for diarrhea, enteritis, typhoid fever, dysentery, and other intestinal diseases.[5] Hanson recognized that the public health nurses had vital roles to bring progressive change; they were the links—often the only links—between policy and the citizens who required uplift and care.

This need in the rural areas was particularly highlighted with the birth of the first county health unit, in Taylor County in 1930. These county health centers were innovations that coincided with the reorganization of the State Board of Health's administration; they promised a robust program of collaboration between the board and county commissioners to meet local public health needs. The law of 1931 to permit Florida's counties to establish their units passed after Taylor County established its own with the help of US Public Health Service funds. Each county health unit would be under the supervision of the state board, with Mettinger supervising all public health nursing requirements for the units. Provisions allowed some smaller counties to join together and necessitated the basic staff of a physician, nurse, and sanitarian to have additional public health training. The units allowed for consolidation at a local level of all health programs administered by cities, counties, schools, and other organizations like the Red Cross. In 1931 Leon County was the second to launch a unit, and within ten years thirty-five units had opened. At the end of World War II in 1945, the total had increased to forty-three. In 1960 St. Johns County established the final unit, completing statewide coverage through county health units. Their development was an opportunity to provide a broad range of health services to communities and respond to local health needs. Central to serving those needs was the role of the public health nurse. In 1930 Taylor County's unit demonstrated the desperate need and the nurses' uphill climb to bring change to a rural community.[6]

The first county health officer, Walton H. Y. Smith (1898–1976), painted a picture of Taylor County as burdened with malaria and hookworm.[7] Sanitation in towns was fairly good in response to the lumber industry's initiatives. Joyce Ely deserves credit for her part in spreading the gospel of health in Taylor County towns, but from the edge of one town to another most country people remained ignorant of preventive medicine and health precautions. Going their separate ways on goodwill tours, the professional public health trio consisting of the health officer, nurse, and sanitarian most often encountered "blank stares and a thinly veiled hostility" to their introductions. Resistance to change had been a constant in Florida's rural places from the time the first public health nurses set out in 1914. "What was good enough for Pappy is good enough for me" was the frequent response.[8] According to Smith, slowly the nurse found her way into the homes, but getting through to the occupants was another matter. One technique with measurable success was to show moving pictures to illustrate the value of screens, privies, and other preventive measures. In one home a mother with a family of "hookwormy children" flatly refused to cooperate. She insisted that "there was no such thing as hookworms, and if there was a moving picture of them it was made up because you couldn't take a picture of something that wasn't."[9] Getting through to this woman obviously required patience, tact, and perhaps creativity in the form of Jule Graves's storytelling technique.

In many ways the rural people tested the trio's perseverance. As the sanitarian assisted with the work of privy building, a different kind of resistance arose. Smith explained, "The beautiful screen doors were kicked out because mamma couldn't get the door opened fast enough to throw out the dirty dish water," and the privies went unused. Smith pointed out one family of eight as a "classic example." Living deep in the county, they were "filled to overflowing with hookworms . . . potbellied and pasty faced." They were too sick for the usual treatment of carbon tetrachloride, so Smith prescribed the new drug hexylresorcinol requiring several stages of treatment as well as the installation of a new privy. But even with "nods and smiles" indicating that the family would use the privy, it remained unused. Finally, Smith learned the reason. The family was so pleased to get their health back they could not "possibly use the beautiful new house that the health unit had built for them for that desecrating purpose."[10] Still, the trio plodded on with educational programs, privy building, hookworm treatment clinics, school programs, and an antimalarial program. Hookworm was indeed a battle when school by school and class by class the specimens most often remained positive. The quinine clinics, too, were misunderstood. People received enough quinine sulfate for the week with instructions to take it prophylactically, but instead they stockpiled the medicine waiting for chills and fever to occur. The trio pressed on until the third year of operation, when Taylor County commissioners decided to discontinue the health unit. They disagreed with the many who believed the unit was strong enough to stand on its own. "They threw out the health unit, lock, stock and barrel and replaced it with a nurse," concluded the disappointed Smith. He bemoaned that the trio "tried to do a good job and succeeded only in being considered expendable and unnecessary."[11]

The reestablishment of the Taylor County health unit in 1936 and in fact, the birth of all the county health units in Florida boiled down to a story of salesmanship.[12] It was imperative that influential citizens of the counties sell the great need to the commissioners; once again the women's groups stepped forward. Leaders of the Florida Federation of Women's Clubs joined with local parent-teacher associations and others to galvanize support. Selling a change in public health

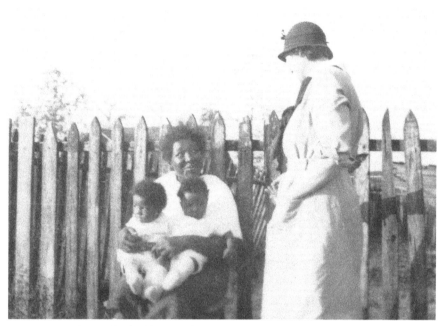

Figure 5.1. A white public health nurse from the Taylor County Health Unit visits an African American mother and her twins, ca. 1936. Courtesy of the State Library of Florida.

operations also required cities with health departments to pool their resources with their counties. The concept of providing better service to schoolchildren was one way to convince school boards that children's needs could be more effectively served with an organized unit than by a nurse working alone. Many local officials quickly saw the benefits a county health unit could bring, but for others, obstacles had to be ironed out. For some it was finding the additional tax money necessary; for others it was the incessant cries of "state medicine" reminiscent of objections to the Sheppard-Towner Act a decade earlier.[13] Still the move to establish a unit in every county was afoot, and in 1936, the same year Taylor County commissioners reinstated that county's unit, the Pinellas County Health Unit opened its doors, revealing a public health nurse's part in selling the concept of efficient public health work to the commissioners.

The public health nurse Martha L. Stetson's (1894–1968) grounding in the public health needs of Pinellas County provides a window into the development of its county health unit. Such needs came to light in 1918. The county's clubwomen employed Stetson's predecessor, Ruth Barnum, to address children's health in schools and become the first county nurse. By the time Barnum retired in 1922, she had proven the dire need for the expansion of public health services. In the absence of a health officer during these early years, the responsibility to improve the program fell upon Stetson, a Red Cross nurse who had served as a US Army nurse from 1918 to 1921. Stetson's family had moved to St. Petersburg in 1913; she was familiar with the area, and her professional skills made her a perfect choice to reach into rural homes, take up the battle against hookworm, malnutrition, impetigo, and granulated eyelids, and verify to the county commissioners the great need for her work.[14]

Her work was always open for evaluation by the county commissioners. Stetson recalled that on one occasion a commissioner demanded to see for himself exactly "what, where and how the public health nurses were spending their time and if they were really 'on the job' in their districts."[15] Although it is unclear what specifically motivated his concern, it coincided with a monetary commitment of $5,000 each by those counties of Florida that were willing to participate in a program initiated by the Rockefeller Foundation International Health Board to support public health nursing and deliver school inspections and other public health services to rural areas.[16] Subsequently, the commissioner began his tour of inspection on a typical hot and humid summer day when Stetson arranged for him to accompany her on her routine tour to visit many rural families. In Pinellas, as elsewhere, there continued to be a high incidence of hookworm among schoolchildren. In some schools more than 50 percent of the children were infected. It therefore fell upon public health nurses to educate parents and children about improving home hygiene and sanitation and to take the initial step toward the diagnosis of the disease by collecting stool specimens during home visits and sending them for laboratory examination. Stetson was accustomed to the long and rugged country roads and the foul odors emitting from the accumulating stool specimens bumping along on the rear seat. The commissioner, however, was not. Stetson remembered that for him it was "an endless day, he made no comment except to say he had had enough and never again would utter a word about another inspection tour!"[17]

The commissioners relied on Stetson's reports to demonstrate the ultimate need to develop the Pinellas County Health Unit. By 1936 her reach had extended throughout the county, drawing in citizens to support welfare programs. In 1927, when nine hundred children lacked clothing to attend school, she encouraged the Junior Service Club, the precursor to the Junior League, to collect clothing donations. In the early 1930s she collaborated with the organization to run the first prenatal and baby clinics. In 1936 she sat alongside Ruth Mettinger on the board of the newly formed Pilots Club, an organization of professional philanthropic women who initiated a fund-raising drive to establish a clinic for African Americans.[18] Stetson's work to establish the clinics fed into the development of the Pinellas County unit and shows her autonomy in the field. She demonstrated how as a Red Cross nurse fired up with patriotism she turned her attention to seek out and serve those in need. She drew in citizen participation, developed community programs, and like Mettinger, strengthened the nursing profession through leadership positions in the Florida State Nurses Association. Stetson epitomized how the public health nurses' work contributed to the organization of county health programs in Florida. They facilitated a new era of community leadership, an opportunity for local governments and citizens to take an active part in health programs, and a base to accelerate the public health nurses' reach into poorly served areas.

Underscoring Inclusion with Caveats

In 1934 the first mobile unit for chest X-rays was a step forward to facilitate the diagnosis of active or suspected cases of tuberculosis, but the continuing battle with the disease presented one of the most pressing problems facing Mettinger and Hanson. "There has always been a great need for someone to go into the home where tuberculosis has one or more victims," noted Hanson, "to teach those afflicted how to conduct themselves so as to be a minimum danger to others, especially young children, who are most susceptible and the ones first to become infected." Twenty years after the first public health nurses began the work in 1914, the high and disproportionate tuberculosis death rate among African Americans continued. Statistics from 1931 show 427 deaths among 1,064,000 white residents and 640 deaths among 442,000 black residents. "The most acute need for visits by public health nurses is in the homes of the colored where there are active cases of tuberculosis," concluded Hanson. "It is for lack of nursing care and prophylaxis that the tuberculosis rate among the colored in Florida is 3.6 times as high as the white rate." It was clear to both Hanson and Mettinger that a robust public health nursing program to address tuberculosis and other health problems requiring preventive services must include African American nurse leaders. "We ought to have several Negro Public Health Nurses on the regular staff," advised Hanson.[19]

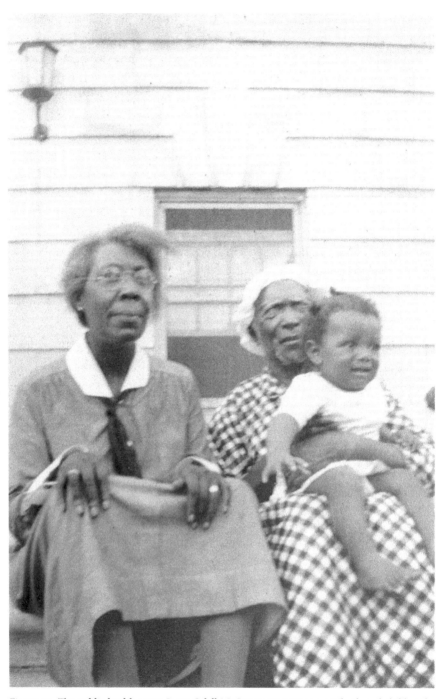

Figure 5.2. The public health nurse Irene Odell McGreen sits next to a midwife and child at the Midwife Institute in Tallahassee, 1933. Courtesy of the State Library of Florida.

The year Mettinger took office there were several black public health nurses who had made their mark in Florida. Rosa Brown was one. Hanson hailed her work in the Okeechobee region as outstanding. After the initial start from the Red Cross, Brown's work continued with a grant from the Julius Rosenwald fund. "We owe the Rosenwald fund a debt of gratitude," noted Hanson.[20] In 1934 "Nurse Rosa Brown" was one of the Board's four black and fourteen white local supervisors of midwives taking responsibility for regular monthly meetings, checking bag equipment, and holding classes. Their race was clearly identified in the board's reports. All supervisors had "R.N." after their names, but as in the earlier reports, the nod to Jim Crow continued. Black supervisors were not afforded the title of "Miss" or "Mrs." One exception, however, slipped through the channels. Brown's counterpart, the midwife supervisor "Nurse I. [Irene] Odell McGreen," who assisted Lalla Mary Goggans with the development of the first midwife institute, appeared on the nursing roster for 1930 without a race identifier. But the possible significance of a step forward was negated when that year all nurses were listed only by first and last names without titles.[21] McGreen went on to become the first public health nurse to join the Leon County health unit when it opened its doors to expand health care services at a grassroots level. Hanson and Mettinger recognized how public health nurses like McGreen and Brown paved the way for others to follow and did so in spite of the wall of segregation that stood so firmly erect in the state. As Mettinger pointed out and Ethel Kirkland would demonstrate, wearing their uniforms was indeed a badge of courage as they continued to work as outsiders within the health system, improving lives in spite of the difference and marginalization inflicted upon them.

An Increase in Nursing Power

When so many people suffered and struggled financially during the Depression, it was one of Mettinger's first tasks to administer a statewide nursing program under the Federal Emergency Relief Act. The program brought relief to Florida's 275 out-of-work nurses and responded to local and county health organizations' requests. Without an accurate account of the number of organizations employing public health nurses, Mettinger's first move was to conduct a survey. Counties, cities, and school boards employed fifty-nine nurses, the newly founded county health units five, the Red Cross four, and other organizations twenty-three, making a grand total of ninety-one nurses. "There is no reason for any organization to look at the Federal Emergency Relief Nursing Service with fear and trembling," Mettinger reassured the health organizations of the state, "wondering how it will function and whether it will disrupt and antagonize the [established] agencies" in the state.[22] She was at the ready to cooperate with all the agencies and provide the necessary supervision of the nurses to best serve the people of Florida. With this distinct aim in mind, she ensured one or more nurses for each county. When many counties had never before had a public health nursing service, she saw the increase in the numbers of nurses as a golden opportunity to build support for the permanency of the service.

After conducting a survey of unemployed nurses, Mettinger assigned one or more of the Federal Emergency Relief nurses to each county and devised a plan to make sure their work was meaningful to themselves as well as to the communities they served. Hospital training was not sufficient for the public health field, Mettinger warned, and she made clear how the field of public health nursing was different.[23] Many Federal Emergency Relief nurses were private duty nurses who entered homes by invitation for specific purposes under the instruction of attending physicians. Families had no voice in the selection of public health nurses, so the nurses had to find ways to diplomatically reach people, as Graves epitomized. Highlighting further differences between private duty and public health nursing, Mettinger made sure the Federal Emergency Relief nurses understood that public health nurses most often worked alone in the field. She explained that the nurses worked with standing orders for treatment and medication endorsed by each county medical society, specifically when no physician was in attendance. But in many counties physicians were never in attendance. To ease them into their work, Mettinger placed the nurses under the wing of district supervisors who had public health training and experience.[24]

Jule Graves, the Southwest District supervisor, promised the federal relief nurses a warm welcome and understanding of the work at the first Federal Emergency Relief Nursing institute held in Tampa.[25] After calling the morning session to order—using a Lysol bottle as an appropriate gavel—she went on to discuss the maternity and infancy program, stressing exhibits, simple methods, and innovations for proper infant care. Mettinger taught the value of the Red Cross Home Hygiene and Care of the Sick classes, and Hanson brought up the need to educate and supervise the midwives of the state.[26] He explained that even though the midwife law had passed in 1931, the State Board of Health was "handicapped" by lack of a penalty clause for "those who persist in practicing without a license."[27] As addressing the problem largely fell on the public health nurses who interacted with the midwives, progress toward change could only be achieved through diplomacy, a skill essential to a public health nurse, as Mettinger earlier pointed out. The institute grounded the federal relief nurses in the basics to contribute to the public health of their assigned communities. Whether they were visiting families on relief, conducting physical examinations of children, or taking the home hygiene classes into schools, Mettinger urged them to prove their worth. She was mindful that when federal funds were withdrawn, it would be important for their work to continue.[28]

"Without the interest of the community, a public health nursing service would soon die," Mettinger noted, encouraging the nurses to strengthen ties with the communities by spearheading the founding of public health nursing councils, organizations consisting of laypeople with the public health nurses acting as the liaisons.[29] Mettinger highly valued these councils to demonstrate a nurse's work and to receive community support. Unless there is "a body back of her, her work loses significance," noted Mettinger. Importantly, the nurse would be "guarded against unjust criticism."[30] The public health councils bore fruit when the Federal Emergency Relief project was discontinued on December 1, 1935, and the number of nurses was reduced by half.[31] Counties had begun to step in with funding, with just three making a head start before Works Progress Administration funding came through in February 1936. The following year Mettinger reported that the growth in the number of public health councils to sixty statewide reflected a confidence in the nursing service. "Fear, indifference and suspiciousness lessened," she noted. During the grim Depression years the councils became advocates for the nurses to procure supplies for the clinics and funds to provide many undernourished children with cod liver oil and milk.[32] When the Works Progress Administration program discontinued in 1939, twenty-nine counties had assumed financial responsibility for the nurses, and other counties promised further commitments. That year the local public health nursing councils morphed into the statewide Public Health Committee, but Mettinger pointed out that it was merely a name change and that activities remained "practically the same." The 1930s had brought stronger partnerships between the public, nurses, counties, and state that contributed to development of the county health units and the means for public health nurses to extend their reach.[33]

By the time the American Public Health Association evaluated the health situation of Florida in 1939, Mettinger had already brought sweeping changes to the nursing program, most specifically to raise the standard of education for white and black public health nurses employed by the state. Through Social Security funds the State Board of Health was able to absorb many of the Works Progress Administration nurses, including the five district supervisors, now renamed "consultants." With the board's nursing personnel reduced from seventy-five to thirty-five, those who could matriculate from a course in public health nursing approved by the National Organization for Public Health Nursing were absorbed into county health units. A major problem in securing qualified personnel was the educational deficiency of many potential hires. Still, Mettinger arranged for those with deficiencies to make them up and for others to seek career advancements with scholarships through Social Security funds. The latter included Grace Higgs, who headed to the Medical College of Virginia, Ethel Kirkland to Lobenstein School of Midwifery in New York, and those who proceeded to Peabody College in Nashville, Columbia University, William and Mary College, and other public health schools.

The reorganization of the Bureau of Public Health Nursing in 1939 set the tone in the following decades to strengthen the county health units. The consultants spent time evaluating how best to meet the needs of citizens and made recommendations to increase the nursing staff, a necessity in tune with the America Public Health Association's recommendation. They found that decentralization secured more community support and interest and built up attendance in clinics. As Mettinger and the nursing consultants acted in an advisory capacity to all the nurses of the state, whether employed by the units or not, monthly reports from nurses in the field indicated the extent of their push to drive the development of the county health centers. They worked relentlessly to eliminate hookworm, conduct Home Hygiene and Care of the Sick classes, and involve local physicians in venereal disease clinics.

In 1940, of a total of 168 public health nurses in the state, 69 worked in county health units. The following year Mettinger reported "rapid progress" of qualified public health nurses, with 19 additional nurses joining county health units. In 1942, with an increased appropriation, a total of 161 nurses were employed in county health units; two-thirds of them met the qualifications, and four of the county supervisors headed for specialized training at Peabody.[34] The American Public Health Association reported that "health services in Florida still have a long way to go before they can meet the needs of the people." The public health nurses under Mettinger's guidance were putting forth their best effort to rectify those needs, but the problem remained for the rural poor. Those counties with a county health unit showed the dire need in those without one.[35]

In the Field

In the latter part of 1936, the State Board of Health inaugurated a Division of Tuberculosis, responsible for establishing tuberculosis clinics in counties. The clinics' success depended on the fieldwork of nurses. As the prime goal of these clinics was to discover early symptoms and eliminate the spread of disease, the consultant Clio McLaughlin was well versed in the cultural mores of the state and well qualified to lead the nursing charge. Earlier she was one of Florida's Sheppard-Towner Act nurses, and she went on to specialize in tuberculosis. Where county health units were established, she instructed the public health personnel and public health nurses in the prevention of tuberculosis, the care of patients with the disease, and the importance of tuberculin testing in schools. Tuberculin skin testing started in 1932, and by 1936 further advances came when X-ray units could be dismantled and moved from clinic to clinic. McLaughlin made it clear that the work of the public health nurses was necessary to precede the clinicians. It was essential that they prepare the district nurses, local doctors, and school boards to support carrying the antituberculosis measures into schools. Then at the end of 1937, when the first sanitarium opened—almost thirty years after Florida's clubwomen first called for its establishment—the public health nurses' work expanded. Along with educational work in schools, preparation for tuberculin testing, and X-raying people came another great responsibility that focused on handling the post-sanitarium patient.[36]

The new state sanitarium proved wholly inadequate to meet the needs of the 10,000 active cases of tuberculosis in Florida. Even though the incidence of tuberculosis was highest among African Americans and the death rate three and a half times greater, the bed capacity of 400 was unevenly distributed, with 300 for white patients and 100 for black patients.[37] A. J. Logie, the director of the Division of Tuberculosis reported concern about the high death rate among the twenty to forty-five-year age group, the wage earners, and the increasing mortality among African Americans. In spite of improved economic conditions, the death rate was not due to more frequent infections but to the fact that once infected the African American population was less resistant to progressive disease. Saying "tuberculosis is curable," Logie energized a new effort to reach the African American and white population, the old and the young and to control the disease by finding cases in the early stages, work that heavily relied upon the public health nurses.[38] Although confining patients in the sanitariums was not cost-effective, without alternatives the state health officer W. A. McPhaul suggested that the answer to the inadequate and unequal provision of sanitarium beds lay with the counties. Escambia County had a sanitarium with a capacity of forty-four beds, twenty-four for whites and twenty for blacks. Those numbers should be the goal in every county, he maintained.[39] By 1943 tuberculosis had become a war problem since many of the men called by the Selective Service were rejected because of infection. Temporary hospital facilities opened and subsequently led to the establishment of more permanent hospitals in the 1950s in Lantana, Tampa, and Tallahassee.[40] With the new drugs streptomycin, para-aminosalicylic acid, and isoniazid, treatment changed, hospital stays declined, and the overall death rate fell. The 1950 death rate was 19 per 100,000; in 1960 the rate was 2 per 100,000.[41]

The subsequent improvement in mortality occurred in spite of the 1939 American Public Health Association criticism of the health situation in Florida and the State Board of Health's response to the high death rate among and lack of sanitarium beds for the African American population. Once again, the American Public Health Association evaluators made the point that "as long as tuberculosis is permitted to continue its ravages in the colored race, the rate among the white population will continue high."[42] Restating and echoing earlier concerns, this report asserted that the "colored maids found in so many homes in Florida" were surely an example of ways the disease spread from the "colored to whites." The report reminded the State Board of Health that "public health recognizes neither color, race nor creed. It must attack communicable disease wherever it exists in the human race."[43] Such a tenet drove Mettinger's guidance of the nursing department, and she clearly pointed it out for readers in *Florida Health Notes*: "The nurses give special attention to the problem of tuberculosis and venereal disease among the colored population."[44]

Grace Higgs exemplified Mettinger's assertion, demonstrating how African American nurses in the field worked to counter local resistance to clinics when people often wrongly asserted that their neighborhoods were tuberculosis-free. For Higgs, fieldwork in Miami began soon after she returned from graduation at Tuskegee School of Nursing in 1935, just as the Labor Day hurricane wiped out the overseas railway in the Keys and killed more than 250 people. This emergency was the only time she worked at a hospital before beginning her thirty-five-year tenure as a public health nurse. She recalled that her later work took her into the outlying rural areas of Dade County "under adverse and even primitive conditions" as well as the segregated communities of Miami. She served in clinics, made home visits, treated pellagra, visited schools, supervised midwives, conducted immunizations, helped to eradicate hookworm, and gained a reputation as a tuberculosis specialist. Higgs encouraged people to take advantage of the mobile X-ray units that traveled the state during the 1940s into the 1960s. If a film showed a shadow or an abnormality, she facilitated the patient's treatment from the health department or a private physician. Like other black nurses in the state, Higgs was highly respected in her neighborhood and served as a role model to young black women not only for the way she conducted her fieldwork but also for her professional achievements. While she worked to break down the barriers of ignorance about health in neighborhoods, she also quietly worked toward breaking down the barriers of race in the nurses' professional associations. Her ultimate goal, quite simply, was to improve people's health and save lives.[45]

Mettinger was clear that fieldwork to locate patients conducted by Higgs and others was the key to finding cases of all communicable diseases and in particular to aid in the war against syphilis. When he became the US surgeon general in 1936, Thomas Parran stepped up the campaign against venereal disease that he initiated when he directed the US Public Health Service Division of Venereal Disease a decade earlier. He declared that one in ten Americans suffered from the diseases, a figure Karen Kruse Thomas has noted was an overstatement, but it drove home his point that the disease was a national problem. The new surgeon general emphasized that "every citizen, North and South, colored and white, rich and poor, has an inalienable right to his citizen's share of health protection" and that a health service must focus on facilitating that right.[46] From the start Parran emphasized health neglect in the South and looked for ways to recruit black doctors and nurses, believing—just as the founding platform of the National Association of Colored Graduate Nurses had advocated in 1908—that black nurses were best suited to see the needs of their people. Then, during World War II, white military recruits tested positive for syphilis at the rate of 48 per 1,000, and the rate among black recruits was 272 per 1,000, figures highlighting the disparities of race, living conditions, and access to medical care.[47] Public health nurses were absolutely essential to follow through with the long, drawn-out, seventy-two weeks of treatment, tellingly dubbed by patients as "them hip shots."[48] Parran went on to actively encourage black women to join the Cadet Nurse Corps during the war, an action that had a profound effect on Florida. After the war, many who had taken advantage of the cadet nursing program joined the public health nursing force of the state. By then, penicillin treatments had streamlined the medical management of venereal disease. In 1947, with the opening of the board's Rapid Treatment Center at Melbourne, a few former cadet nurses found work.[49]

In response to Parran's directives, Mettinger drove his policy home at a grassroots level. She made it clear that nurses were the vital link to get the message across to the community at large where many were fearful that the "pox" or "bad blood" was "punishment for their sins." A public health nurse was particularly "fitted because of her many contacts with the public," Mettinger noted. First, the nurses needed to free their own minds of ancient taboos and bring their own knowledge of the diseases, methods of prevention, and treatments up to date. "No one has a better opportunity to assist in locating patients in the early stages than the public health nurse," Mettinger insisted. With the nurse's up-to-date knowledge of facilities for indigent cases, "she may by means of objective or subjective symptoms, suspect and seek out cases." Mettinger clarified the earlier claim made by Joseph Porter, the first state health officer, that the nurse is often a patient's most trustworthy friend. Similarly, Mettinger wrote, "Many secret fears are confided in her, in her role as a trusted advisor."[50] She warned against professional chauvinism and prejudice and instead demanded the "humanizing, individualizing and personalizing of the nurses relations with syphilitics." If patients could see they were not "cogs in the wheel" they would be encouraged to go to the clinics.[51] Furthermore, she insisted that the nurses' work expand to educate the general public and civic organizations.[52]

The public health nurses' fieldwork to address venereal disease included a concentrated effort within the maternity program to ensure the best chance to secure the "inalienable right of every unborn child to be born free from syphilis."[53] *Florida Health Notes* painted a picture of the urgency of addressing the matter. "Five out of six babies born of *untreated* syphilitic mothers are born dead or diseased," it reported. In the late 1930s on average there were still 1,500 stillbirths in Florida every year, with syphilis a leading yet easily preventable cause.[54]

In an attempt to reduce the number of stillbirths and congenital syphilitics, a negative result in a Wassermann test was one condition imposed upon midwives before they could obtain a license. Maternity clinics routinely conducted the Wassermann test, but private physicians who did not want to offend patients with the blood test posed problems. It was a question of reeducation, argued Mettinger, positioning herself again to trumpet Parran's redefinition of syphilis as a communicable illness like tuberculosis.[55] People needed to understand that venereal disease was not a "moral deviation to be prevented by scorn and cured by penitence, but rather a community health problem," she affirmed.[56]

During the 1940s and into the 1950s, as syphilis, tuberculosis, and maternal and infant deaths continued to take their greatest toll among African Americans, the State Board of Health continued to cite ignorance and poverty as the main contributors to these conditions. *Florida Health Notes* ran an article, "Ignorance and Quacks Take Heavy Toll among Negroes: Units Attacking Problem," stating that "most negroes have not been taught what to do" and ignored the efforts made by the public health nurses but that "those who have, are usually without funds to carry out the teaching."[57] The purpose of the article was to emphasize the importance of the county health units and to credit those counties with efficient units for making progress to "correct these problems."[58] It was the public health nurses radiating from the units, working alongside midwives, conducting fieldwork, and finding cases, who were largely responsible for this progress. Another *Florida Health Notes* article promoting the Rapid Treatment Center stated that alongside other fieldworkers, "public health nurses relentlessly pursued 'contacts' over the State."[59] Yet, the "Ignorance and Quacks" article missed an opportunity to speak out specifically in favor of the fieldwork of the nurses; instead it condemned African American communities. "Too often negroes are the prey of unscrupulous persons, many times persons of their own race," the statement read. The call for "the interest of conscientious people, both white and colored who are in a position to help them" spoke directly to the space the public health nurse—black or white—had sought to occupy since the nurses first stepped into the communities in 1914.[60]

Ethel Kirkland's Role in the Midwife Program

In his reflection in 1980 on Florida's midwifery program, Dr. Wilson T. Sowder, the state health officer from 1945 to 1969, brought to light the extent to which

Ruth Mettinger was a standard bearer for all nurses. In doing so he offered insight into the obstacles black nurses encountered during Jim Crow.[61] He also discussed the larger-than-life personality of Jule Graves and the "quiet, modest and very competent person" Ethel Jones Kirkland, who worked alongside Graves as the state midwife teacher.[62] After Graves retired in 1947, Kirkland ran the program through the remaining years of Jim Crow, until in 1971 she declared that she was close to working herself out of a job.[63]

Sowder began by stating facts: in the 1930s and 1940s it was unheard of to campaign against unfair salary practices in the era of "encrusted traditional discrimination."[64] He confirmed the outrage Mettinger had felt toward the racial policies employed by state officials in the 1920s, her embrace of the more just policies of the Red Cross, and her intent to make a change. She believed black nurses should not only be employed by the State Board of Health but also receive the same grade and salary as white nurses. According to Sowder, she took action. It required mobilizing the white nurses to support her claim for hiring Kirkland. Sowder added, "And she gained her point." Looking back at the discrimination from a viewpoint after the civil rights movement, Sowder concluded that such unfair practices were "almost unbelievable now." He wrote, "Ethel was such a perfect lady and who never asked for any favor even this one, that it was impossible to oppose such obvious justice for her."[65] But Kirkland's silence in the face of discrimination and other demeaning practices during her tenure at the State Board of Health actually highlighted the racial undertones that shrouded her work with the midwifery program.

True to the tradition of Jim Crow, the board's annual report for 1936 underscored Kirkland's race by recording her first position in the Bureau of Public Health Nursing without the title "Miss." Perhaps Mettinger believed it was a small step forward to list Kirkland alongside the eight supervisors, but being listed as "Nurse Ethel Mae Jones" marked her difference.[66] (She married Tom Kirkland shortly thereafter.) If Kirkland had no choice but to overlook the slight, she saw how the position itself gave her the power to enact her goals. She had seen what was needed in the midwifery program and what she wanted to do when she began her tenure in the rural areas of north Florida as a federal relief public health nurse.[67] Her race opened doors to the black communities, and her position as the state midwifery teacher gave her the authority to enact the board's policy. Though Jim Crow compromised boarding facilities and travel, her mobility was outstanding. She traveled the state, staying in counties for two to three weeks at a time, checking and rechecking those midwives who were licensed and those who were not, holding group meetings, observing deliveries, and advising on postpartum care. From the start Mettinger praised Kirkland's efforts and the impact the black midwife teacher made when she mirrored the race of the people she sought to serve. "She accomplished a great deal and enabled this Bureau to have a more accurate record of the midwives, and has assisted reduction of maternal death rate by observing more closely those midwives who are not conducting their work properly," Mettinger reported.[68]

It took Graves and Kirkland an exhaustive effort to reduce the number of registered midwives from approximately 1,100 in 1936 to 575 in 1939. Graves had conducted one-day midwife institutes, and Kirkland had spent two to three months at a time to visit various county health units to give intensive instruction to midwives and follow up on their cases. Overall the establishment of the units allowed for closer supervision of midwives and provision of prenatal care. Midwives brought their patients into clinics and often remained with them through examinations. But if doctors were becoming more interested in the welfare of these patients in some counties and if, as Mettinger put it, "people were becoming educated for a physician delivery," there were still problems, particularly in the rural areas. Country folk could not pay the fee for a physician even if one was available. Hospitals could not care for all indigent cases, and private physicians could not be expected to offer free care. Quite simply, the rural population made it impossible to eliminate the midwife altogether.[69]

The 1940s opened with Kirkland, now a Lobenstein-trained nurse-midwife, initiating an effort to replace the elderly, retired midwives with handpicked high school graduates who were interested in training as midwives under the board's guidance. In Mettinger's words, since Kirkland's return from New York she had "filled a great need in the state." As a vital part of the Graves-Kirkland team, she brought her own unique means to interact with the black midwives and prospective midwives.[70] The new generation of midwives would be "far better to carry on this work," Mettinger reported. Her overall plan included replacing "the granny midwife with nurse-midwives who [could] more intelligently carry the phase of the work." The plan moved forward when Lille Mae Chavis and two other black public health nurses working in health units of rural counties undertook a six-month course in midwifery. Upon returning to their units they supplemented Kirkland's statewide supervision by taking full charge of midwife work in those counties.[71] As other health unit nurses were not so well prepared to oversee the midwives of

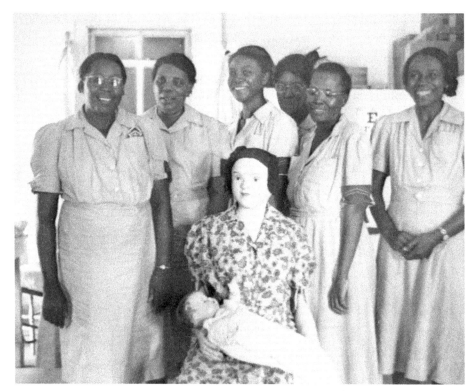

Figure 5.3. A new generation of midwives in training poses in 1949 with "Miz Chase," the mannequin made by Jule Graves. Courtesy of the State Library of Florida.

their counties, Graves held one-day midwife institutes to teach them methods of supervising the midwives. Kirkland concentrated on the midwives and spent one to four months at the units to get closer one-on-one observations of them at work and to offer practical advice and teaching on an individual basis.[72] Still, difficulties remained, as Kirkland pointed out. Mettinger reported that the "problem to which the better midwives are seeking a solution is that of securing adequate medical assistance with complicated deliveries or hospitalization."[73]

Throughout the war years, after Graves's retirement in 1947 and through the 1950s, Kirkland made her rounds to supervise midwives individually and in groups by making field visits to individual midwives and conducting institutes to reach many at one time. Her push to persuade elderly midwives to retire and replace them with younger ones continued.[74] Of 461 in 1948, one was eighty-four years old, two were seventy-nine, and twenty-seven were seventy-three. The ages of the remaining midwives ranged between twenty-five and fifty-eight.[75] The midwives' numbers were gradually decreasing. The 1952 figure of 365 was 58 fewer than the year before, indicating the retirement of the elderly midwives as well as the additional hospital beds for maternity patients and the private physicians' acceptance of referrals.[76] Yet some of the county units' health officers recognized that midwives continued to have a vital place in some places. If they observed that additional midwives were necessary, Kirkland was there to interview and train the candidates.[77] Conversely, by 1960, eleven county health officers had declared that midwives were no longer needed and discontinued their licensure, resulting in the total number dropping in the state to 228 licensed midwives.[78]

Kirkland could be encouraged that the maternal and infant death rates had improved since 1935, largely reflecting the success of the midwife program even though there were racial disparities. Statistical evidence from Bureau of Maternal and Child Health in 1960 showed this improvement. In 1935 the white maternal death rate per 10,000 live births was 73 and the nonwhite 117. Twenty-five years later, in 1960, the rate of white maternal deaths dropped to 2 per 10,000 and the nonwhite to 12. But the statistics remained a concern, especially when some maternal deaths in 1960 were classified as "preventable." Similarly, the white infant death rate per 1,000 live births for 1935 was 50.2, whereas the nonwhite rate was 88.0. Again, twenty-five years later, in 1960, the nonwhite infant death rate had dropped to 23.8, while the nonwhite rate was still high, at 45.7. The leading cause of infant death was prematurity, but with the improved prenatal care for the mother, the increased availability of incubators for home use, and supervision of the infants' care at home, the State Board of Health expected further decline of the infant mortality rate.[79]

Kirkland insisted that an important part of the midwifery program was to teach midwives to accompany their patients to the prenatal clinics operated by the county health units. By 1960 the clinics, primarily for the indigent, made it possible that by State Board of Health reckoning every mother in Florida could secure prenatal care. Whether delivery was attended by a midwife or a physician, most clinic attendees expected to deliver at home. Overall hospitalization plans were not forthcoming in many counties, giving credence to Higgs's earlier assertion that African American women expecting routine deliveries could not choose hospital deliveries. Therefore, midwives could only be eliminated if local physicians and hospitals were able to care for indigent patients. In 1962, the year before Mettinger retired, Kirkland continued to plan and conduct educational programs for the 203 midwives of the state.[80]

Kirkland's work reflected that finally, tradition and superstition had been replaced by modern childbirth procedures—whether practiced in homes or hospitals—and the maternal and infant mortality rates reflected the reform. The midwifery program was not without its critics. Debra Ann Susie has argued that the State Board of Health measured the program's success not by the upgrading of the midwives' skills but by eliminating their practices. She contends that the focus on elimination was a reflection of the state's control over midwives and a goal that did not respect the midwives or their work.[81] Such a view led to calls for a new era of lay midwifery that began in Florida in the late 1970s. But that view did not take into consideration the broader implications of race during the Jim Crow era—the lack of choice for African American women but also the lengths the public health nurses like Kirkland had to go to circumvent racial mores to reduce the maternal and infant death rate to save people's lives.

Again, it was Sowder who highlighted the quiet manner in which Kirkland responded to an internationally publicized racial incident when Kirkland and Deborah Coggins, the health officer for Madison County, sat together for lunch at the local Hotel Madison. Kirkland had come to Madison to instruct recent high school graduates in midwifery skills. When classes began on August 20, 1956, Coggins was eager to learn of their progress and arranged to meet Kirkland at her only time available, during the lunch hour. Approximately two weeks later the fireworks exploded. Two years after the US Supreme Court's *Brown v. Board of Education of Topeka* decision, rumors turned to cries that Coggins was in favor of desegregation and school integration and was even "sleeping with black men in a Tallahassee motel on a weekly basis."[82] The news spread as the local press publicized the commissioners' meetings as being infused with ugly calls for Coggins's resignation.

Even though she was not without supporters including Sowder, who recommended that the commissioners take "no further action," Coggins lost her job.[83] Across the nation and even the world, headlines screamed out when the Associated Press picked up the story: "Health Officer Faces Loss of Job after Lunch with Negro" and "Florida Health Officer Fired for Lunching with Negro."[84] Governor LeRoy Collins reported that he "was sick about it," declaring that the furor was a "by-product of the passions aroused by efforts to coerce integration of the people against the will of the people."[85] Coggins's stormy response to her firing emblazoned the reports. She stormed out of the meeting, calling the commissioners "fools and cowards" for not directly stating that she was ousted as a direct response to her lunch with Kirkland. "Cowards! Lady Gets Last Word on Firing," reported the *Dallas Morning News*,[86] but her firing had a ripple effect on her supporters as well by weakening health services and eliminating the midwives' classes that Kirkland was hoping to strengthen. Yet it was Coggins, not Kirkland, and not consideration of the benefits of training midwives but the maintenance of social mores that were the focus of the news reports and a subsequent scholarly article.[87]

Soon after Coggins's firing, Sowder was met with questions when he attended a conference in New York, but none addressed Kirkland. "I asked why none had thought to ask what had happened to the black public health nurse. . . . They said, well, what happened to her? I replied that nothing had happened to her." Yet the striking silence toward the experience from Kirkland's perspective was only confirmed by Sowder himself. Evidently, he admired "her dignified behavior . . . and for passing up an opportunity to get national recognition," noting that no newspaper ever got a quote from her.[88] But he never mentioned the incident to her, and when he broached the subject at a Christmas party, she thought he was referring to the midwife program and was pleased with the compliment.[89] Perhaps for Kirkland the incident was but a more magnified and publicized version of racial slights that she faced in her everyday life—reaction would detract from her mission.

And so, at the dawn of the civil rights movement, in the words of Betty Hilliard, a nurse instructor at the University of Florida, Ethel Kirkland, as always, "kept her cool" when faced by such racial slights in the course of her work.[90] In the early 1960s Hilliard invited her to the university to talk to students about the midwife program. "We took her to the cafeteria at lunch time and they [the cashiers] stopped us. 'She can't come in here.' And I said, 'well she is our guest.' So the cashier thought about it for a little bit" and came up with a solution. "Maybe if one of you gets in front of her and the other ones get behind her, really close so that everybody looking at her knows you are with her, it will be all right. You could try that." It seems Kirkland had no choice. "Ethel was okay . . . I don't know how," asserted Hilliard.[91] Reflection upon the compromise of Kirkland's civil rights gave Hilliard and Sowder pause. To be sure, for Kirkland and other black nurse leaders of Florida, living with such discrimination day in and day out strengthened their fight for their civil rights in nursing. It was one way to face the statewide and nationwide discrimination.

A Meeting of the Minds

Throughout her administration, Ruth Mettinger insisted that the public health nurse's uniform mattered. It mattered to the public health nurses across the state, white and black, and it mattered to the communities they served. Importantly it mattered to the young black women growing up in the state and seeking role models. One recalled admiring a public health nurse riding her bicycle and "looking so good in her uniform." Another remembered a public health nurse working in the community wearing a red-lined navy cape. "I wanted to be just like her," this nurse recalled.[92] The role models, in turn, lived up to expectations not only to carry their public health work into the black communities but also to establish equitable standards within their professional organizations.

Ethel Kirkland, Rosa Brown, Bessie Hawes Smalley, Grace Higgs, and others finally realized their goal of forming the Florida State Association of Colored Graduate Nurses in 1935 and proceeded to pursue plans toward integration of the professional associations.[93] They were aptly assisted by Mettinger, who spoke at their conventions and made a lengthy proposal for their inclusion during the 1942 convention of the Florida State Nurses Association: "Negro nurses are given membership in the National Organization for Public Health Nurses; Negro Welfare workers are given membership in the National Conference of Social Workers; Negro nurses are allowed to enroll in the Red Cross Nursing Service," she argued. "There is no law in this state prohibiting Negro nurses from becoming members of the Florida State Nurses Association."[94] Mettinger's motion carried that "qualified Negro nurses be permitted membership in the State organization."[95] The decision to admit black nurses in 1943 made Florida's state nurses association one of the first in the South to integrate.[96] In 1947 Higgs, president of the Florida State Association of Colored Graduate Nurses, was the first African American to sit on the Florida State Nurses Association Board of Directors but as a courtesy member, without vote or voice.[97] This silence would not be tolerated by her successor, Mary Elizabeth Carnegie, dean of the School of Nursing at A&M College in Tallahassee from 1945 to 1953. Florida State Nurses Association records make Carnegie's leadership qualities clear: "Those who know Mrs. Carnegie realize that when issues were raised in her presence, she was not one to 'have no voice.' She spoke out with forthrightness and vigor."[98]

Carnegie had taken up the challenge of reorganizing Florida's first baccalaureate-granting nursing school to further the careers of all black nurses in the state, a goal she shared with Mettinger.[99] Succeeding Higgs as president of Florida's black graduate nurses association in 1949, on a motion also made by Mettinger, Carnegie's vocal leadership bore fruit.[100] She became the first African American nurse elected to the board of directors for the Florida State Nurses Association, making it the first state association of the nation to include black board members.[101] That same year Carnegie was at the forefront of the march toward integrating the national organization as well. At the National Association of Colored Graduate Nurses convention in Louisville, Kentucky, Carnegie and her counterparts voted to dissolve their organization after barriers were finally removed for black nurses' membership in the American Nurses Association. Since nurses joined the American Nurses Association through their state associations, in those southern states that denied black nurses membership the nurses could join the American Nurses Association individually. In 1951 the National Association of Colored Graduate Nurses legally dissolved, but the problems of segregation, salary differentials, inequalities in job opportunities, and other matters continued to concern black nurse leaders in spite of the American Nurses Association platform promising "full participation of minority groups in association activities . . . and the elimination of discrimination in job opportunities, salaries and other working conditions."[102] In theory Carnegie had initiated a new chapter for black nurses in Florida, an achievement that was thoroughly endorsed and facilitated by Mettinger, but in practice the state and district meetings and even work and everyday life continued to be exercises in racial discrimination.

The Cadet Nurse Corps of World War II had opened the door for more women to train as nurses, and in the postwar scene white nurses could look forward to choices for their career path, but black nurses faced limitations. For many it was the differences within hospitals that made institutionalized racism so hard to bear. Thelma Anderson Gibson's experience was typical. She expressed her objection to her status as an outsider within the health care facility by fighting back. At Jackson Memorial Hospital she aspired to a position in the operating room but found it was out of bounds for black nurses. The only position available to her was on "Colored II," a surgical floor where the differences between black and white nurses were strictly observed. "Colored nurses could not be head nurses," she explained. She noted further, "Colored nurses could not teach whites even though Jackson's white nursing students had to come to the Colored wards for experience."[103] Although she was told to call herself and her counterparts "Nurse" and not "Miss" or "Mrs.," she challenged the rule, leading the older nurses to fear she would be fired. "It was a matter of pride," Gibson told the director when she was called to the office for a reprimand. "I was taught to call myself Miss and my patients Mr. and Mrs."[104] As a consequence of such prejudice many newly trained nurses like Gibson preferred public health work. Gibson embraced the field, furthered her education at Teachers College, and became a role model for others to follow her path. In 1964, the year of the Civil Rights Act, she was the first African American assistant supervisor of nurses at the Dade County Health Unit.[105] Gibson's career path reflected a turning point for black nurses, one that Mettinger had worked for and supported throughout her administration. By the time she retired, the movement for change that had brewed for decades promised a more just future for the nurses, but their work in the wake of Jim Crow also assured them continuing struggles to serve Florida's disadvantaged population.

Mettinger's leadership in Florida during the Jim Crow era demanded strength and fearlessness and a team of like-minded professional women. Surgeon General Parran argued that such qualities were still necessary even a century after Florence Nightingale paved the way to reform nursing practice. "Among the reasons why the light from the lamp of Florence Nightingale shone far was because she was known to be perfectly ready to throw it at anybody who stood in the way of righteous progress," he wrote. In the public imagination, Nightingale lived on as a saint. But Parran reminded readers that "she achieved those good works because she had a clear eye, a pungent tongue and a heart so filled with wrath at needless suffering that she spared no one, no matter how highly placed, or who might be responsible for it."[106] For Mettinger, Brown, Foote, Reid, Goggans, Graves, Kirkland, and other public health nurses, the suffering they encountered in Jim Crow Florida demanded righteous progress not only for the white and black, urban and most especially rural people they served but also for themselves. They all must have been perfectly ready to throw Florence Nightingale's lamp at so many of Florida's obstacles. Instead they shone that lamp to navigate through the cultural mores of the state—to do the good works of saving lives in Florida—and were often the only ones who could.

Conclusion

Tracing Footprints from the Past

An informative 1990s poster distributed by the Florida Department of Health and Rehabilitative Services warned people to be aware that tuberculosis was highly contagious and had made a comeback.[1] The message targeted minorities, who were disproportionately affected, particularly African American men between the ages of twenty and forty-four years. The poster warned people to be aware of the signs and seek treatment that was easily accessible by contacting the local health department. If by including the image of Irene Odell McGreen as the "main line of defense" in the 1930s the health authorities intended to illustrate how far the treatment had come in sixty years, why then was there such a racial disparity existing between the tuberculosis rate of African American and whites? This was a question that state and national health authorities addressed in the 1990s and continued to research into the new millennium. Several studies that considered the poor access to health care and the great social and economic disadvantages concluded that the problems had many facets and required further study.[2] The historian David McBride, however, is blunt. The depth of his twentieth-century study of tuberculosis and the AIDS crisis among African Americans has led him to urge the medical community to consider the racist paradigms that continued to obscure the cause of epidemics, encumber treatment, and impede prevention.[3] His words have relevance to the consequences of this study. The inclusion of McGreen, a black nurse, to offer a message to the black community indicates that the racial division cementing people into categories was magnified during Jim Crow and yielded severe implications in health care policy. McBride points out that the racial

In The 1930s Public Health Nurse McGreen Was Your Main Line Of Defense Against TB

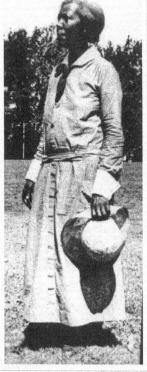

Once nearly extinct, tuberculosis is making a comeback - especially in Florida.

TB is highly contagious -- and it affects a disproportionate number of minorities, especially black males, ages 20 - 44.

Tuberculosis can be cured with proper treatment. Be alert to the symptoms:

- *Persistent cough or fever*
- *Shortness of breath*
- *Night sweats or fatigue*
- *Coughing up blood.*

You can schedule a TB test and get more information on turberculosis by contacting your local health department.

Today, It's A Simple Call To Your Local Public Health Unit

DEPARTMENT OF HEALTH AND REHABILITATIVE SERVICES

A message from the Florida Department of Health and Rehabilitative Services.

Nurse McGreen is believed to have been one of Florida's first African American public health nurses. Photograph courtesy of the Florida State Archives.

Figure C.1. The inclusion of a historical image of the public health nurse Irene Odell McGreen in this 1990 health poster illustrates the long battle to fight tuberculosis. Courtesy of the State Library of Florida.

bias in health care policy in place during the twentieth-century treatment of tuberculosis and syphilis was repeated during the 1980s AIDS epidemic. A contemporary poster would far better serve the public if it reflected Mcbride's conclusion that racial discrimination was so closely intertwined with tuberculosis and AIDS that they cannot be addressed as separable problems.[4]

There was another underlying message in that poster, one that called for a reflection of the past work of the public health nurses. The inclusion of Mc-Green as the "main line of defense" portrayed a public health nurse who was a bridge—and the only one—to bring health incentives to her community. On another level, therefore, it seems that the Department of Health and Rehabilitative Services' choice to picture McGreen's fight against tuberculosis in the 1930s was a conscious effort to smudge the racial undertows that kept African American public health nurses as outsiders though they worked within the State Board of Health. Regardless of what the racial discrimination in the workplace might mean for McGreen, the Department of Health and Rehabilitative Services obviously intended to honor her by capturing her image and recalling her past. The small print in passive voice at the base of the poster, however, indicates the department's uncertainty regarding that past: "Nurse McGreen is believed to have been one of Florida's first African American public health nurses." This vagueness actually included the history of Florida's white nurses as well. The present study adds certainty to the work of McGreen and her counterparts, black and white, who emerge from the shadows of the historical record.

The public health nurses of Jim Crow Florida addressed the ongoing battle against diseases and for the well-being of people by navigating cultural roadblocks and discriminatory health policies. These nurses found ways to physically and mentally reach people who were marginalized from modern health initiatives. Examples abound. Each decade offered case studies that illuminated the nurses' agency and highlighted the illnesses and health experiences facing Floridians before the nurses took action. Irene Foote found the two tubercular sisters sleeping in the same bed and instructed the father on how to make an outside sleeping porch. Rosa Brown took the matter of the deplorable living and health conditions in the "Negro section" of West Palm Beach into her own hands to bring about much-needed change. And Jule Graves offered examples of folk lore and practices in her work with midwives. Her unique methods often saved the lives of mothers and infants who were subjected to harmful practices. The nurses like Foote, Brown, and Graves often utilized their own directives to individually or collectively enact and reinforce policies that were critical to their work even as they were inseparable from racist ideology and professional prejudice. Moreover, in this book I bring out what the poster did not: professional discrimination targeted black nurses like McGreen and challenged them to face the double-edged sword in their ongoing fight to save lives.

If McGreen and other black nurses of her era had no choice but to work as outsiders within the system during Jim Crow, after the civil rights movement emerged, many black nurses demanded further change. For some of the nation's black nurse leaders, the dissolution of the National Association of Colored Graduate Nurses and the promise for change that came with their acceptance into the American Nurses Association fell short. These black leaders were no longer willing to accept an outsider status within the American Nurses Association that was not allowing them leadership positions or influence on policy decisions. It was not just a question of their professional needs; their underlying concern was to address the health needs of the black communities in Florida and across the nation.[5]

During the 1970 American Nurses Association convention, held in Miami, black nurses caucused to discuss common goals and concerns. The nurses were "concerned about and accountable to black people in a special way," Elizabeth Carnegie reported. They "felt there was a need for them to articulate the health needs of the black community, as well as provide equal access to and mobility within the health care system."[6] In effect the black nurses voiced similar concerns to those that drove the founding of the National Association of Colored Graduate Nurses six decades earlier as Rosa Brown clearly articulated them. "We could see the needs of . . . our people as no one else could," she stated.[7] Following the civil rights activism of the 1950s and 1960s, once again concerned black nurses took a step toward addressing the advancement of black communities' health by unifying black nurses nationally and in 1971 by inaugurating the National Black Nurses Association. The founding principles have driven the ideals of the association into the new millennium to the present day: "To serve as a national body to influence legislation and policies that affect black people and work cooperatively and collaboratively with other health workers to this end."[8] In Florida members of the National Black Nurses Association took up the mantle of their predecessors to address the consequences of the social construction of health and chart their path forward as the state embarked on a new era of bureaucratic public health practice.[9]

The Upshot of Bureaucratization

In 1970 the arrival of a northern-based public health nursing leader, Dolores Wennlund (1922–2010), coincided with the aftermath of changes from the dissolution of the State Board of Health the previous year. Wennlund found that the picture of Florida's public health nursing contrasted sharply with her northern experiences. Born in the Bronx and armed with a master of science degree in public health, a long career as a public health nurse with the New York Health Department, and work as a lecturer in public health at Adelphi University, Wennlund initially relocated for health reasons. Soon responding to the state's salubrious weather, she accepted a position as a public health nursing consultant in southwest Florida and took the opportunity to bring her northern-based initiatives to the state. She developed school health programs, established nurse advisory committees, and conducted workshops throughout the state. Her leadership skills stood out at a time of turmoil for the state leadership in public health nursing.[10]

Wennlund's early work in Florida overlapped with the complications that had arisen within the state and counties' health administrations and resulted in the general marginalization of public health nurses. By the late 1960s tensions that had mounted between the local health departments and the State Board of Health over the allocation of federal funds came to a head. Legislators considered organizational changes and finally took steps to abolish the State Board of Health. Once the board was abolished in 1969, structural changes ensued. The Division of Public Health Nursing became a section within the Department of Health and Rehabilitative Services, and the director's title changed to that of administrator. According to Wennlund, the many layers of nurse leadership stemming from a local level with the county health units and public health agencies amounted to a step backward in the professionalization of public health nursing. Jane Wilcox, the state nursing administrator, was most concerned with the loss of control overall and particularly in the educational qualifications of the nurses. The problem "caused alarm and consternation precipitating the resignation of Jane Wilcox in 1974," stated Wennlund.[11] It seemed that Ruth Mettinger's earlier push for the public health nurses' educational requirements amounted to little consequence.

The history of public health nursing in Florida is a prime example of what Karen Buhler-Wilkinson refers to as a "false dawn." The public health nursing profession failed to fully deliver the promise of economic security and professional independence that were the founding principles that drove the leadership of public health nursing in the second and third decades of the twentieth century. Some of Florida's early leaders who tried to move the profession forward stood out: Irene Foote in 1916, Laurie Jean Reid in the 1920s, and Ruth Mettinger thereafter, at first wearing two hats, one for the Red Cross and the other for the State Board of Health. Their leadership, however, was strapped as public health nursing evolved and nurses secured employment with different types of public and private agencies. Nurses themselves were unable to establish a fully unified state body in spite of the leaders' intent. Nurses in Florida and other states failed to interconnect into a powerful national body. Then changes in the hospital-based system of medical care and marginalization of the public health nurse within the broad health care system stymied professional growth.[12] Wennlund found that Florida's "public health nurses did not have a large role in the public health field." She lamented, "The nurses were taken for granted by the doctors, by everyone, even themselves."[13]

Wennlund began her fifteen-year term as Florida's public health nursing director in 1974 to lead in an era that corresponded with further reorganization and restructuring of Public Health Nursing Services and a move toward the total bureaucratization of public health. While she restored the requirement for a baccalaureate degree as a minimum qualification for community health nurses and established policies and procedures necessary for the changing times, the bureaucratization led her to reflect on the lack of control of nursing services, an outcome surely epitomized in Buhler-Wilkinson's term "false dawn." By the end of the century, some county administrators reduced the authority of nursing directors, some deleted the position, and some field-nurse supervisors were appointed and supervised by non-nurse supervisors. "Case finding," Wennlund noted, a core public health nursing service that Florida's public health nurses excelled at during Mettinger's administration, "was seldom heard during the '80s." No longer assigned to neighborhood sections, no longer making house calls, the public health nurses instead undertook heavy clinic workloads that in Wennlund's words "inhibited the creativity and freedom . . . to be effective case finders, to be responsible for and familiar with a community and its needs."[14] For Wennlund, the health care bureaucracy undercut the personal touch of nurses.

Reckoning with the Past: Midwives in Changing Times

A large part of the public health nurses' work that transitioned the midwife problem into the midwife program offers an understanding of the social construction of health that carried footprints through Wennlund's era as director to the continuing complexity of unequal health care and the broader societal view of racism today. Laurie Jean Reid's prophesy in 1923 that it would be "years and years" before the women of the state could rely on a trained obstetrician for their maternity care was correct.[15] "Decades and decades" would have been more correct, with the caveat that a trained obstetrician would be available only for those who could pay the obstetrician and hospital fees or even a doctor for a home delivery. Midwives provided an essential service particularly to the African American community and the rural areas throughout Jim Crow times and beyond. But until the 1980s, securing a midwife for delivery was not a question of choice for most women. Thus, the cultural mores of the midwifery program laid the groundwork for the consequences it entailed.

In the early 1970s Ethel Kirkland believed she was close to working herself out of a job.[16] While there was a decline from the 191 licensed midwives in 1964 to just 57 a decade later, those practicing midwives, as the 1972 annual report indicates, continued to be vitally needed in a few areas of the state.[17] The decline reflected changes brought on by the entitlement programs that established the delivery of medical care for eligible candidates. An example is the Hospital Survey and Construction Act of 1946, known as the Hill-Burton program for its sponsorship by Senators Harold Burton and Lister Hill. In return for accepting federal funds for construction and modernization, hospitals were obligated to provide free or low-cost medical care for those in need.[18] By the 1970s, however, attorneys for the poor continued to seek justice for their clients from those hospitals failing in their commitment to provide charity care.[19] Still, hospital desegregation and Medicaid enabled most black women to deliver their babies in hospitals, but questions remained concerning a black women's choice for delivery, especially in the rural areas. According to the midwife Johnnie Seeley, many black women preferred to engage a midwife: "It may have been for the simple reason that they don't have any midwives is why they went [to a hospital]. . . . They don't go because they prefer to go. A lot of them would rather stay home, but they just have to go."[20]

In the wake of the second wave of feminism, a grassroots movement led mostly by middle-class white women demanded a greater choice in birthing practices. Their insistence energized a new generation of white midwives to battle Florida's legislature, obtain licenses, and secure the revival of midwifery and home births. The issue was complicated. Earlier, official reports utilized the term "granny midwives" to separate the traditional midwives' identity from the registered nurses who, like Kirkland, had received additional maternity training to become certified nurse midwives. In 1972 there were ten certified nurse midwives in Florida working at the county health units to provide maternity and family planning services. Jane Wilcox, the state nursing administrator, said that "barriers to the fullest utilization of nurse-midwives in Florida" remained, and the elimination of these barriers "was essential to the provision of adequate maternity services in Florida."[21] Instead, the barriers grew even though by 1980 there were only twenty-five "granny" or "lay" midwives in the state. One problem centered on the vital statistical reports that grouped all midwives' deliveries together although the certified nurse midwives attended births in hospitals and the lay midwives in homes. Together the midwives delivered a total of a little more than 2.5 percent of all births, a proportion that had increased from 1 percent in 1975.[22] The increase came down to a question of choice and power and reflected the need for a broader understanding of racial, class, and professional hierarchies. The new lay midwives demanded and won greater control over their practices with the passage of the Midwifery Practice Act of 1982. Yet barriers remained for the Certified Nurse Midwives triggering professional jealousy. They were obliged to "work under a doctor." On the other hand, lay midwives "could function independently."[23] Wennlund confirmed that the difference "never ceased to irk" the professionally trained nurse-midwives.[24] In increasing numbers, however, these highly qualified nurses were becoming a part of the broader feminist movement whose advocates objected to the power of the paternalistic medical profession and to the reining in of their autonomy.

In their thrust to legitimize the profession, the modern-day lay midwives hailed their predecessors, the granny midwives, for their important service to the community but in the process downplayed the racism and cultural condescension of the public health nurses and the health departments, as Christa Craven and Mara Glatzel point out.[25] After 1980 the impetus to collect the elderly granny midwives' own accounts grew, but missing in the discussion and interpretation of them is important context that must include and go beyond acknowledging the presence of racism and cultural chauvinism within the board's program. The public health nurses who drove Florida's midwifery program offer a more complicated history and one that explores the historical contingency centered on the dire figures of maternal and infant mortality. Granny midwives were not remembered for the mortality and morbidity records; rather, the modern-day midwives sought to "reclaim their roots in catching babies" and replicate practices like those of Augusta Wilson, who maintained that childbirth at home was "better. 'Cause when a woman have a baby at home, she have more privileges. See, she can walk. . . . A woman can move around during her labor. . . . But you see in hospital, no quicker than you get there they put you in a bed and let you stay there by yourself."[26] The midwives practicing during Jim Crow facilitated the modern-day midwives' changing the climate of midwifery in Florida but in the process highlight the reason for the critical need to explore the historical contingency of Florida's midwife program in those times.

Other consequences come to light that pose questions. Could insights into the Jim Crow era add to the conversation on the disparities of modern-day health outcomes in maternity care? Today, African American women experience worse birth outcomes than any other major ethnic group. Black infants are more than twice as likely as white infants to die within their first year, due largely to premature birth, low birth weight, or birth defects.[27] This disparity has triggered many discussions in the popular media drawn from scholarly studies to examine racial differences and stress factors that contribute to the birth outcomes.[28] Recent studies conclude that perceived racism during childhood and throughout life contributed to poor birth outcomes.[29] Indeed, the present examination of the stress factors linking racism with poor birth outcomes throughout the Jim Crow era offers a grounding to help explore the continuing problems of today.

If conscious and thoughtful action to change policy is called for, can the pioneer public health nurses offer clues that might add to the discussion? For example, after the long road of exclusion to hospitals for childbirth, their ultimate inclusion led many black women to feel isolated within the institution. Like many of her counterparts, the midwife Wilson spoke out about the advantages of home deliveries versus hospital ones, but underneath her colorful language is a layer of distrust and dismay. She noted, "They going on about their business, or there the nurse over there with her feet in the chair reading. The doctor home laid up with his legs crossed reading a book. And there you in the room by yourself."[30] In her own words Wilson described her perception of the impersonal attitudes of hospital staff, reflecting a barrier that had the potential to reverberate and disconnect women from modern health care even as the aftermath of civil rights, women's rights, and health care rights movements brought new visions of inclusion. As I have explored in this study, the public health nurses who worked during Jim Crow sought to alleviate the many layers of disconnection to bring the promise of contemporary medicine to those who were left out. Race complicated their reach, but through it all they were the bridges to connect with people physically and just as importantly, mentally, to correct misunderstandings, allay fears, conduct community meetings, teach Home Hygiene and Care of the Sick classes, educate midwives, hold clinics, and more. The nurses' interplay and interconnections with the midwives, country people, and others illustrated their commitment to meet the cultural challenges of Florida. Their work holds significance in contemporary America, where maintaining healthy lives for all Americans is a matter of meeting the nation's deep-rooted cultural challenges.

Finally, from the time the first three public health nurses set out to serve people on foot or by train, automobile, and boat, the public health nurses of Florida looked for ways to improve people's lives. Racial laws, custom, and innuendo complicated their delivery of care, but through it all, their basic tenet was to prevent disease and deaths and improve people's health. Such health care challenges, interwoven with social justice concerns, whispered in circles throughout the twentieth century, into the twenty-first century, and to the present day. In 1992 Wennlund concluded that "public health nursing had gone many miles" in support of prevention, yet there still remained too many who needed public health services but were left out. For Wennlund the resolution was obvious. While "the disenfranchised . . . the poor, the disadvantaged, the vulnerable populations exist," she concluded, "there will always be the need for a public health nurse to find them, to awaken the community to their needs, to provide the nursing services they need, and to guide them through the system so that they can receive other services necessary for their health and welfare."[31]

In 2019, as lawmakers work toward replacing or improving the Affordable Health Care Act, many believe the most vulnerable in society will be without health care. Some leaders in public health have long asserted that more than ever a sense of community and the goals of social justice will fall upon today's public health nurses, the community health nurses.[32] My hope is that an understanding of the work of the public health nurses during the Jim Crow era will inform today's community health nurses and add to their conversation as they work toward connecting their social action with health policy, a necessity in caring for Florida's diverse and vulnerable population groups.

Notes

Introduction: Opening a New Profession for Women in Florida, 1914 to 1964

1. Laurie Jean Reid, "Square Pegs in Round Holes," *Florida Health Notes* 21, no. 10 (October 1929): 128. When Laurie Jean arrived at the State Board of Health, her title was director of the Bureau of Child Welfare, a position that included the supervision of public health nursing. The bureau was officially named the Bureau of Education and Child Welfare. On April 19, 1926, the name of this bureau changed, and Reid's title became director of the Bureau of Child Hygiene and Public Health Nursing. Henry Hanson, "State Health Officer's Report," in *State Board of Health of Florida Thirty-Third Report: A Decade in Public Health 1923–1932 Inc.* (Jacksonville: State Board of Health, 1933), 4. Hereafter this report is cited as *Decade in Public Health*.

2. Thomas Parran, "Public Health Marches On," *Florida Health Notes* 30, no. 6 (June 1938): 88.

3. "State Worker Arrives Here," *St. Petersburg Times*, July 21, 1923, 7.

4. Rosa L. Williams [Brown], extracts of speech to the International Council of Nurses convention, Cologne, Germany, August 1912, in Elvira F. Beckett, "Of Interest to Nurses," *Journal of National Medical Association* 5, no. 4 (1913): 270–272. The speech is printed also in Rosa L. Williams [Brown], "The Social Work of the Coloured Nurse," *British Journal of Nursing* (November 23, 1912): 412–413, and noted in Adah B. Thoms, *Pathfinders: A History of Progress of Colored Graduate Nurses* (New York: Garland, 1985), 108.

5. Edward H. Beardsley, *A History of Neglect: Blacks and Mill Workers in the Twentieth-Century South* (Knoxville: University of Tennessee Press, 1987), 28.

6. For Susan M. Reverby and David Rosen's argument see Laurie B. Green, John McKiernan-Gonzalez, and Martin Summers, introduction to *Precarious Prescriptions: Contested Histories of Race and Health in North America*, ed. Green, McKiernan-Gonzalez, and Summers (University of Minnesota Press: Minneapolis, 2014), ix.

7. Green, McKiernan-Gonzalez, and Summers, introduction, viii-xii. Keith Wailoo, for example, focuses on sickle cell disease in Memphis to examine the interconnections of a disease that affected people of African descent with race, medicine, and American society. Going beyond the city, he explores the changing experience of the disease among the people who

suffered from it. For Wailoo, the interplay and interconnections uncovered how the cultural construction of the disease affected funding and patient care. *Dying in the City of the Blues: Sickle Cell Anemia and the Politics of Race* (Chapel Hill: University of North Carolina Press, 2001). See also Andrea Patterson, "Germs and Jim Crow: The Impact of Microbiology on Public Health Policies in Progressive Era American South," *Journal of the History of Biology* 42, no. 3 (Fall 2009): 529–559; Christine Ardalan, "Racialized Medicalization in the United States and Its Borderlands from the Early 19th through the 20th Century," *Journal of American Ethnic History* 35, no. 3 (Spring 2016): 92–98.

8. For nurses' roles as conveyers of information and intermediaries see Karen Buhler-Wilkinson, "False Dawn: The Rise and Decline of Public Health Nursing in America, 1900–1930," in *Nursing History New Perspectives, New Possibilities*, ed. Ellen Condliffe Lagemann (New York: Teachers College, 1983), 94; see also Ryan Johnson and Amna Khalid, *Public Health in the British Empire: Intermediaries, Subordinates, and the Practice of Public Health, 1850–1960* (New York: Routledge, 2012), 3–4.

9. Robyn Muncy, *Creating a Female Dominion in American Reform, 1890–1935* (New York: Oxford University Press, 1991), 115–120; Molly Ladd-Taylor "'Grannies' and 'Spinsters': Midwife Education under the Sheppard-Towner Act," *Journal of Social History* 22, no. 2 (Winter 1988): 256; Susan L. Smith, *Sick and Tired of Being Sick and Tired: Black Women's Health Activism in America, 1890–1950* (Philadelphia: University of Pennsylvania Press, 1995), 139.

10. Patricia Hill Collins, *Black Feminist Thought: Knowledge, Consciousness, and the Politics of Empowerment* (New York: Routledge, 1990), 10–11.

11. Karen Buhler-Wilkinson, "Guarded by Standards and Directed by Strangers: Charleston, South Carolina's Response to a National Health Care Agenda, 1920–1930," in *Enduring Issues in American Nursing*, ed. Ellen Baer, Patricia D'Antonio, Sylvia Rinker, and Joan E. Lynaugh (New York: Springer, 2002), 168.

12. Mary Sewell Gardner, *Public Health Nursing*, 3rd ed. (New York: Macmillan, 1938), 268.

13. Buhler-Wilkinson, "Guarded by Standards and Directed by Strangers," 165–179.

14. Steven J. Hoffman, "Progressive Public Health Administration in the Jim Crow South: A Case Study of Richmond, Virginia, 1907–1920," *Journal of Social History* 35, no. 1 (Autumn 2001): 175–194.

15. Elna C. Green, introduction to *In Black and White: An Interpretation of the South*, by Lily Hammond, ed. Elna C. Green (Athens: University of Georgia Press 2008), xiii.

16. Karen Kruse Thomas, *Deluxe Jim Crow: Civil Rights and American Health Policy, 1935–55* (Athens: University of Georgia Press, 2011), 11; John Duffy, *The Sanitarians: A History of American Public Health* (Urbana: University of Illinois Press, 1992), 226.

17. "National Association of Colored Graduate Nurses Minutes," August 18, 1914 (1908–1917), vol. 1, reel 1, National Association of Colored Graduate Records, 1908–1951, Schomberg Center for Research in Black Culture, Jacksonville Public Library, Jacksonville, FL (hereafter NACGN Records).

18. Williams, speech to International Council of Nurses.

19. Laurie Jean Reid, "Public Health Nursing: A Factor in Child Welfare," *Florida Health Notes* 14, no. 8 (December 1922): 135.

20. Arlene W. Keeling, *Nursing and the Privilege of Prescription, 1893–2000* (Columbus: Ohio State University, 2007), 8; Darlene Clark Hine, *Black Women in White: Racial Conflict*

and Cooperation in the Nursing Profession, 1890–1950 (Bloomington: Indiana University Press, 1989), 101.

21. Medical inspection of schoolchildren, instituted in Boston in 1894, was already well established in Europe. In 1837 France had begun supervising the health of children in schools. This was followed by Belgium, Germany, England, Sweden, Russia, Austria-Hungary, and further afield in Egypt, the Argentine Republic, and Chile prior to 1894. Gardner, *Public Health Nursing*, 352.

22. Although following the lead of New York, many cities made the mistake of employing only doctors to perform medical inspections of schoolchildren. They discovered that the "best method was to use the nurse for routine inspection with a doctor as a consultant, and follow-up in the homes of children, done by nurses." Minnie Goodnow, *Outlines of Nursing History*, 6th ed. (Philadelphia: W. B. Saunders, 1938), 362.

23. Gardner, *Public Health Nursing*, 39.

24. Muncy, *Creating a Female Dominion*, 46.

25. Muncy, *Creating a Female Dominion*, 39, 47.

26. In Victor Robinson, *White Caps: The Story of Nursing* (Philadelphia: Lippincott, 1946), 29.

27. Gardner, *Public Health Nursing*, 41; Harriet R. Feldman and Sandra B. Lewenson, *Nurses in the Political Arena: The Public Face of Nursing* (New York: Springer, 2000), 36.

28. Hine, *Black Women in White*, 101.

29. Gardner, *Public Health Nursing*, 41–43; Feldman and Lewenson, *Nurses in the Political Arena*, 36.

30. Lillian Wald to Jacob H. Schiff, December 1910, in Lavinia L. Dock, *History of American Red Cross Nursing* (New York: Macmillan, 1922), 1213. The American Red Cross Public Health Nursing Service began as the American Red Cross Rural Nursing Service in 1912, three years after the professional Red Cross Nursing Service was established as a reserve for the Army and Navy Corps and a corps of nurses ready for disaster relief work. In 1913 the American Red Cross Rural Nursing Service expanded as the American Red Cross Town and Country Nursing Service and in May 1918 was renamed the American Red Cross Bureau of Public Health Nursing. In 1921, during the American Red Cross Nursing Service reorganization, the Bureau of Public Health Nursing was renamed the American Red Cross Public Health Nursing Service. Portia B. Kernodle, *The Red Cross Nurse in Action 1882–1948* (New York: Harper and Brothers, 1949), 51, 63, 73, 131, 246.

31. "Town and Country Nursing," file 494.1, box 34, record group (RG) 200; "Florida," file 159.1, box 264, RG 200, American National Red Cross (hereafter ANRC Records), National Archives and Records Administration, College Park, MD (hereafter NARA).

32. For excerpts of Dock's speech see "13th Annual Convention," *American Journal of Nursing* 10, no. 11 (August 1910): 902.

33. For a reproduction of the program "The First Annual Convention of the State Graduate Nurses Association of Florida," January 29–31, 1913, see Karleen Gillies, *Sunshine and Breezes: A Brief History of the Florida Nurses Association, 1909–1984* (Orlando: Florida Nurses Association, 1984), 10–11.

34. The following is a partial list to offer context to Florida's organization: New York was the first to form a state association, in 1901, the same year as Illinois and Virginia. In 1902

North Carolina and New Jersey followed. In 1904 Louisiana formed a state organization, followed by Tennessee in 1905, Kentucky and Texas in 1906, Georgia and South Carolina in 1907, and Mississippi in 1911. Minnie Goodnow, *Outlines of Nursing History*, 6th ed. (Philadelphia: Saunders, 1938), 459.

35. "A Quarter Century of Service," *National News Bulletin: Official Organ of the NACGN* 11, no. 2 (June 1948), publications file 1, box 3, reel 1, NACGN Records.

36. M. Elizabeth Carnegie, *The Path We Tread: Blacks in Nursing Worldwide*, 3rd ed. (New York: National League of Nursing Press, 1995), 79–81; Hine, *Black Women in White*; S. Smith, *Sick and Tired*.

37. Margaret Humphreys, *Yellow Fever in the South* (Baltimore: Johns Hopkins University Press, 1992), 120; Margaret C. Fairlie, "The Yellow Fever Epidemic of 1888 in Jacksonville," *Florida Historical Quarterly* 19, no. 2 (October 1940): 95–108; William M. Straight, "The Yellow Jack," *Journal of Florida Medical Association* 58, no. 8 (August 1971): 31–47.

38. Humphreys, *Yellow Fever in the South*, 125.

39. On the founding of the State Board of Health see William J. Bigler, "Public Health in Florida—Yesteryear," *Florida's Journal of Public Health* 1, no. 3 (May 1989): 4; Albert V. Hardy and May Pynchon, *Millstones and Milestones: Florida's Public Health from 1889*, Monograph Series, no. 7 (Jacksonville: Florida State Board of Health, 1964), 8–18; Wilson T. Sowder, "Recollections of the 100 Year Struggle for Better Health in Florida," part 1 [1888–1950], *Journal of Florida Medical Association* 76, no. 8 (August 1989): 683–688.

40. Hardy and Pynchon, *Millstones and Milestones*, 9-29; Bigler, "Public Health in Florida Yesteryear," 5–6; Carroll Fox, "Public Health Administration in Florida," *Public Health Reports* 31, no. 22 (June 2, 1916): 1359–1363. Fox is identified as "Surgeon, United States Public Health Service."

41. John Duffy, *The Sanitarians: A History of American Public Health* (Urbana: University of Illinois Press, 1992), 3.

42. Joseph Y. Porter, "The Real and False in Sanitation," *Florida Health Notes* 1, no. 9 (March 1907): 2.

43. Porter, "Real and False in Sanitation," 2.

44. William A. Link, *The Paradox of Southern Progressivism, 1880–1930* (Chapel Hill: University of North Carolina Press, 1992), 7.

45. Jessie Wheeler, "Report of District Public Health Nurse," in *State Board of Health of Florida Twenty-Eighth Annual Report, 1916* (Jacksonville: January 1, 1917), 157.

46. George Pretty, interview by Viola B. Muse, November 9, 1936, in Federal Writers Project, *Slave Narrative Project*, vol. 3, *Florida*, p. 273, Anderson–Wilson (with combined interviews of others), https://www.loc.gov/item/mesn030 (hereafter *Slave Narrative Project*).

47. Rebecca Hooks, interview by Pearl Randolph, January 14, 1937, in *Slave Narrative Project*, 171.

48. Charlotte Martin, interview by Alfred Farrell, August 20, 1936, in *Slave Narrative Project*, 165–167.

49. The caption is on the back of the photograph *Portrait of an Unidentified Male Midwife*, ca. 1933, black-and-white photoprint, 5 × 3 inches, State Archives of Florida, Florida Memory, https://www.floridamemory.com/items/show/44605.

50. Grace Higgs, interview by the author, August 18, 1997, Miami.

51. Linda Shopes, "Oral History and the Study of Communities: Problems, Paradoxes, and Possibilities," *Journal of American History* 89, no. 2 (September 2002): 588–598.

52. Hardy and Pynchon, *Millstones and Milestones*, 3–7; Samuel Proctor, "Prelude to the New Florida, 1877–1919," in *The New History of Florida*, ed. Michael Gannon (Gainesville: University Press of Florida, 1996), 266–286; Michael Gannon, *Florida: A Short History* (Gainesville: University Press of Florida, 1993), 53–76; Henry F. Becker, *Florida: Wealth or Waste?* (Tallahassee: Florida State Department of Education, 1953).

53. Charlton W. Tebeau, *Florida: From Indian Trail to Space Age* (Delray Beach, FL: Southern, 1965), 56–57.

54. Lalla Mary Goggans, "The Wonderful Years of Working with Mothers and Children," 1972, box 37, MSC 330, American College of Nurse-Midwives Records 1910–1999, National Library of Medicine, Bethesda, MD (hereafter ACNM Records).

55. Hardy and Pynchon, *Millstones and Milestones*, 6.

56. The historian C. Vann Woodward notes that after 1887 many southern states adopted Jim Crow laws on their statute books: Florida in 1887, Mississippi 1888, Texas 1889, Alabama, Arkansas, Georgia, Kentucky, and Louisiana 1890. Woodward, *Origins of the New South 1877–1913* (Baton Rouge: Louisiana State University Press, Littlefield Fund for Southern History, University of Texas, 1999), 211-212.

57. Wali R. Kharif, "Black Reaction to Segregation and Discrimination in Post-Reconstruction Florida, *Florida Historical Quarterly* 64, vol. 2 (1985): 161–173.

58. Samuel Kelton Roberts Jr., for example, has explored how the language of science directly connected tuberculosis to segregated housing in Baltimore. *Infectious Fear: Politics, Disease, and the Health Effects of Segregation* (Chapel Hill: University of North Carolina Press, 2009). See also David McBride, *From TB to AIDS: Epidemics among Urban Blacks since 1900* (Albany: State University of New York Press, 1991).

59. For conditions in North Carolina, South Carolina, and Georgia see Beardsley, *History of Neglect*, 12.

60. John C. Gramling, "The First Charity Hospital in Dade County Florida," Dade County Hospital Association, n.d., Midwifery file, William M. Straight M.D. Collection, RG 6040, Florida International University Special Collections and University Archives, Miami (hereafter Straight Collection).

61. Fox, "Public Health Administration in Florida," 1360.

62. Green, McKiernan-Gonzalez, and Summers, introduction, viii-xii.

63. McBride, *From TB to Aids*, 10.

64. Patterson, "Germs and Jim Crow," 533.

65. Adams held that the ability toward self-government was originally passed down from the fifth-century and sixth-century Teutonic tribes of the German forests and carried to Britain. The Teutonic seed was responsible for the development of superior English institutions, and thereafter, in the seventeenth century, it was passed on to the New England forests of North America, where it prospered and proliferated. This hereditary chain, however, could only pass through the white race's "pure blood lines." Glenda Elizabeth Gilmore, *Gender and Jim Crow: Women and the Politics of White Supremacy and Jim Crow in North Carolina, 1996–1920* (Chapel Hill: University of North Carolina Press), 67–68; Peter Novick, *That Noble Dream: The Objectivity Question and the American Historical Profession* (New York: Cambridge University Press, 1995), 87.

66. John David Smith, "Scientific History at the Johns Hopkins University," *Pennsylvania Magazine of History and Biography* 115, no. 3 (July 1991): 421–426.

67. John Duffy, particularly his chapter "Bacteriology Revolutionizes Public Health," in *The Sanitarians: A History of American Public Health*, 193–204; Nancy Tomes, "Spreading the Germ Theory: Sanitary Science and Home Economics, 1880–1930," *Women and Health in America*, 2nd edition, ed. Judith Walzer Leavitt (Madison: University of Wisconsin Press, 1999), 596–611.

68. Patterson, "Germs and Jim Crow," 531.

69. James B. Crooks, *Jacksonville after the Fire, 1901–1919: New South City* (Jacksonville: University of North Florida Press, 1991), 61.

70. Roberts, *Infectious Fear*, 5–6.

71. Charles E. Terry, "Report of City Health Officer," in *Jacksonville, Florida, Annual Report of the Board of Health for the Year 1911* (Jacksonville: City Council, 1912), 6.

72. Terry, "Report of City health Officer," 37.

73. McBride, *From TB to Aids*, 10.

74. Williams, speech to the International Council of Nurses.

75. Fox, "Public Health Administration in Florida," 1385.

76. Fox, "Public Health Administration in Florida," 1385.

77. McBride, *From TB to Aids*, 10; Patterson, "Germs and Jim Crow," 555.

78. David McBride has noted that during World War I, two and a half times more black soldiers required treatment for tuberculosis than white soldiers; the most prevalent disease among black soldiers, however, was syphilis. McBride, *From TB to Aids*, 34. World War I statistics concerning the health of black soldiers in comparison to white soldiers was addressed by black physicians of Tuskegee Institute and summed up in an editorial to energize health campaigns: "Let us as physicians and laymen, work together to wipe out our high percentage of venereal infection. . . . There must be a campaign inaugurated and pushed, by leaders of both races, against segregating the colored population to the worst sanitary location in the city." Editorial, *Journal of National Medical Association* 11, no. 3 (July-September 1919): 107–108. In Florida, the state's Tuberculosis Association had taken up what the executive secretary Homer W. Borst argued was an urgent matter when deaths from tuberculosis equaled the deaths in battle. He spoke to the citizens of Miami's "Colored Town," introducing a new initiative—white and black public health nurses to address the disease in the city and among the returning soldiers, black and white. *Miami Herald*, September 13, 1918, 8. For further details see "Tuberculosis Clinic to Be Established in Miami at an Early Date," *Miami Herald*, May 27, 1919, 3; "Taking up the Fight against Tuberculosis," *Miami Herald*, June 6, 1919, 7. On establishment of the Florida Tuberculosis and Health Organization in 1916 see Bigler, "Public Health in Florida Yesteryear," 11.

79. McBride, *From TB to Aids*, 33.

80. Precautions included notification and registration of all infected people coming into Florida, disinfection of houses where people with tuberculosis had stayed, and a caution to readers not to allow consumptive persons to mingle with guests at resorts. Porter's policies are recapped in "Public Health in the 1890s," *Florida Health Notes* 59, no. 7 (July 1967): 296.

81. Harriet Beecher Stowe, *Palmetto Leaves*, facsimile reproduction of 1873 edition (Gainesville: University Press of Florida, 1999), 122.

82. John A. MacDonald, "Plain Talk about Florida for Home and Investments" (Eustis, FL: J. A. MacDonald, 1883), 5.

83. L. C. Manni, "History of Tuberculosis in Florida," *Journal of the Florida Medical Association* 73, no. 4 (1986): 306.

84. "Words to Freeze the Soul," *Tampa Tribune*, April 27, 1909, 5. Many advertisements appeared in other Florida and national newspapers, such as in the *Belleville* (IL) *News Democrat*, October 9, 1909, 2; and *Aberdeen* (SD) *American,* April 2, 1909, 7.

85. Thelma Peters, *Miami 1909, with Excerpts from Fannie Clemens Diary* (Miami: Banyan, 1984), 89.

86. Manni, "History of Tuberculosis in Florida," 305–306.

87. It was not until 1915 that the legislature authorized a Bureau of Vital Statistics and allowed for the appointment of the first State Board of Health vital statistician; Hardy and Pynchon, *Millstones and Milestones*, 27. The reporting of deaths and later the reporting of births were important areas where clubwomen and the public health nurses stepped in to assist local doctors.

88. In Manni, "History of Tuberculosis in Florida," 305–306.

89. Hardy and Pynchon, *Millstones and Milestones*, 23.

90. Nancy A. Hewitt and Suzanne Lebsock, introduction to *Visible Women: New Essays on American Activism*, ed. Hewitt and Lebsock (Urbana: University of Illinois Press, 1993), 2.

91. Irene R. Foote, "Report of District Public Health Nurse," in *State Board of Health of Florida Twenty-Eighth Annual Report, 1916*, 149.

92. Barbara Melosh, *The Physician's Hand: Work, Culture, and Conflict in American Nursing* (Philadelphia: Temple University Press, 1982), 125–126; Susan M. Reverby, *Ordered to Care: The Dilemma of American Nursing, 1850–1945* (Cambridge/ New York: Cambridge University Press, 1987), 110.

93. Conversely, in her study based in Appalachia, Sandra Lee Barney discusses the relations between clubwomen and public health workers; she notes that public health nurses employed by women's clubs were stymied from obtaining too much authority by their subordination to both the clubwomen and the physicians. Barney, *Authorized to Heal: Gender, Class, and the Transformation of Medicine in Appalachia, 1880–1930* (Chapel Hill: University of North Carolina Press, 2000), 107–110.

94. Muncy, *Creating a Female Dominion*, xii.

95. Mary Church Terrell, "Greetings from the National Association of Colored Women," cited in *Roots of Bitterness: Documents in Social History*, ed. Nancy Cott, Jeanne Boydston, Ann Braude, Molly Ladd-Taylor, and Lori D. Ginzberg (Boston: Northeastern University Press, 1996), 406–408.

96. Cott et al., editorial note, *Roots of Bitterness*, 406.

97. On March 10, 1908, the Florida State Federation of Colored Women's Clubs formed in St. Augustine. Lavonne Leslie, ed., *The History of the National Association of Colored Women's Clubs, Inc.: A Legacy of Service* (Bloomington, IN: Xlibris, 2012), 322. Mary Bethune was president of the Florida Federation of Colored Women's Clubs (1917–1925), the Southeast Federation of Colored Women's Clubs (1920–1925), the National Association of Colored Women (1924–1928), and the National Council for Negro Women (1935–1949). Audrey Thomas McCluskey and Elaine M. Smith, eds. *Mary McLeod Bethune: Building a Better World; Essays and Selected Documents* (Bloomington: Indiana University Press, 2001), 132, 287. See also Maxine

D. Jones, "Without Compromise or Fear: Florida's African American Female Activists," in *Making Waves: Female Activists in Twentieth-Century Florida*, ed. Jack E. Davis and Kari Frederickson (Gainesville: University Press of Florida, 2003), 270–293.

98. Paul Ortiz, afterword to *Old South, New South, or Down South? Florida and the Modern Civil Rights Movement: Towards a New Civil Rights History in Florida*, ed. Irvin D. S. Winsboro (Morgantown: West Virginia University Press, 2009), 220–238; Charlton W. Tebeau's chapter "Boom-Bust-Hurricane Twenties" in his book *A History of Florida* (Coral Gables, FL: University of Miami Press, 1971), 378–392; William W. Rogers, "Fortune and Misfortune: The Paradoxical Twenties," in *The New History of Florida*, ed. Michael Gannon (Gainesville: University Press of Florida, 1996), 287–303.

99. The Red Cross leadership campaigned to develop its image as a "teacher and rescuer, fund raiser and benefactor, organizer and social conscience." Patrick F. Gilbo, *The American Red Cross* (New York: Harper and Row, 1981), 32.

100. In 1936 the State Board of Health Division of Public Health Nursing became the newly organized Bureau of Public Health Nursing. The agency remained a bureau until 1946, then became a division again, the Division of Public Health Nursing within the Bureau of Local Health Services. In 1960 it became the Public Health Nursing Section and in 1980 Public Health Nursing Services.

101. Henry Hanson, "Decade in Public Health 1923–1932 Inc.," in *Decade in Public Health*, 10.

102. Parran, "Public Health Marches On," 87.

103. Parran, "Public Health Marches On," 88.

104. "Public Health Nursing" section, *What Is a County Health Department?* special issue of *Florida Health Notes* 65, no. 7 (July 1973): 177.

105. Ruth Mettinger, "Balancing a Program," *Florida Health Notes* 34, no. 9 (1942): 107.

106. Mettinger, "Balancing a Program," 107.

107. Jack E. Davis, introduction to *Making Waves: Florida Female Activists in Twentieth-Century Florida*, ed. Jack E. Davis and Kari Frederickson (Gainesville: University Press of Florida, 2003), 1–6.

108. Laurie Jean Reid, "Child Hygiene and Public Health Nursing: Conclusions," *Florida Health Notes* 22, no. 1 (January 1930): 6.

Chapter 1. Waking Up Communities and Seeking Out the Sick in Town and Countryside, 1914 to 1917

1. Williams [Brown], "The Social Work of the Coloured Nurse," 412.

2. Williams [Brown], "The Social Work of the Coloured Nurse," 412–413. See also Beckett, "Of Interest to Nurses," 270–272; A. B. Coles, "The Howard University School of Nursing in Historical Perspective," *Journal of National Medical Association* 61, no. 2 (March 1969): 110; "National Association of Colored Graduate Nurses Minutes," August 18, 1914 (1908–1917), vol. 1, reel 1, NACGN Records.

3. Crooks, *Jacksonville after the Fire*, 50–57; Terry, "Report of City Health Officer," 4–5.

4. Crooks, *Jacksonville after the Fire*, 53; Ellen Lowell-Stevens, "Report of Health Department Civics Committee," in *Florida Federation of Women's Clubs Yearbook, 1909–1910* (Lakeland: Florida Federation of Women's Clubs, 1910), 43 (hereafter *FFWC Yearbook*).

5. Terry, "Report of City Health Officer," 4–5.

6. Federated in 1898, the Woman's Club of Jacksonville reported 278 members in 1909–1910, enabling it to expand its outreach in philanthropic and charitable matters. Jessie Hamm Meyer, *Leading the Way: A Century of Service G.F.W.C. Florida Federation of Women's Clubs, 1895–1995* (Lakeland: GFWC Florida Federation of Women's Clubs), 18, 29.

7. In Gillies, *Sunshine and Breezes*, 10–11. Foote is listed as one of State Graduate Nurses Association's five board members.

8. In "Legalizing Crime in Florida," *Florida Health Notes* 9, no. 1 (January 1914): 9.

9. Grace L. Meigs cites the 1913 statistics from a 1917 publication by the Children's Bureau, titled "Maternal Mortality from All Conditions Connected with Children," in *The American Midwife Debate: A Sourcebook on Its Modern Origins*, ed. Judith Barrett Litoff (Westport, CT: Greenwood, 1986), 61.

10. Florida was finally admitted to Death and Birth Registration Areas in 1919 and 1924, respectively. "The Model Ordinance for the Registration of Births and Deaths," *Florida Health Notes* 9, no. 7 (1914): 123; "Admission of States to Death and Birth Registration Areas," in *Children and Youth in America: A Documentary History*, vol. 2, *1866–1932*, ed. Robert H. Bremner (Cambridge, MA: Harvard University Press, 1971), 965.

11. In Jacksonville a total of ninety-four stillbirths were delivered by midwives and forty-eight by physicians. Terry, "Report of City Health Officer," 27.

12. Susan L. Smith, "White Nurses, Black Midwives, and Public Health in Mississippi, 1920–1950," in *Women and Health in America*, 2nd edition, ed. Judith Walzer Leavitt (Madison: University of Wisconsin Press, 1999), 446.

13. For the correspondence between the midwives, Assistant State Health Officer Hiram Byrd, and Joseph Porter see "Midwifery," *Early Florida Medicine Exhibit*, Florida Memory, n.d., https://www.floridamemory.com/exhibits/medicine/midwives/.

14. Judith Barrett Litoff, "An Enduring Tradition: American Midwives in the Twentieth Century," in *The American Midwife Debate: A Sourcebook on Its Modern Origins*, ed. Litoff (Westport, CT: Greenwood, 1986), 7.

15. In "Legalizing Crime in Florida," 9.

16. "State Health Board Shows a Grave Evil," *Tampa Tribune*, December 17, 1913, 15.

17. In 1913 Jacksonville's statistics indicate that midwives attended 849 of the 1,632 births. Of the 191 stillbirths, midwives had attended 119 women. The report downplayed the high physician statistic by reporting that "only" 72 stillbirths were conducted by physicians. "The Midwife and Infant Mortality," *Florida Health Notes* 9, no. 3 (March 1914): 49.

18. "Better Florida Babies: State Board of Health Writes about Care That Babies Receive," *Morning Sentinel*, Orlando, November 18, 1914, 2.

19. Crooks, *Jacksonville after the Fire*, 54.

20. Crooks, *Jacksonville after the Fire*, 54; "Legalizing Crime in Florida," 9; "Midwife and Infant Mortality," 48–49.

21. St. Augustine was the first to follow Jacksonville's lead with a city ordinance to control midwifery. "St Augustine, FLA: Health Officer, Public Health Nurse, and Sanitary Inspector; Appointment, Powers, and Duties (Ord 32. Aug. 1. 1916)," *Public Health Reports, 1896–1970* 31, no. 37 (September 15, 1916): 2528.

22. Jean Waldman Shulman, "Introducing Rosa L. Brown, an Historical Red Cross Nurse," *American Red Cross: Nursing Matters Past and Present* (Spring 2014): 4–5.

23. "Miss M. A. Allen's Great Work," *Washington Bee*, August 26, 1911, 1; "Florida Federation of Colored Women's Clubs Hold Interesting Session, *Freeman* (Indianapolis), July 3, 1915, 3; "Take Care of the Babies," *Tampa Tribune*, September 14, 1913, 21.

24. Minutes, Annual NACGN Meetings, 1917, 1920, and 1921, NACGN Records; B. J. Sessions, *A Charge to Keep: Brewster Hospital, Brewster Methodist Hospital, Brewster Hospital School of Nursing, Brewster-Duval School of Nursing, 1901–1966*, (Jacksonville, FL: Brewster and Community Nurses Alumni Association, 1996), 15, 138–139.

25. "State Board of Health Bulletin," *Tampa Tribune*, September 14, 1913, 21. Allen is not mentioned by name in the news article.

26. Fox, "Public Health Administration in Florida," 1385.

27. Charles Harris Wesley, *The History of the National Association of Colored Women's Clubs: A Legacy of Service* (Washington, DC: National Association of Women's Clubs, 1984), 283.

28. Jacob U. Gordon, *Black Leadership for Social Change* (Westport, CT: Greenwood, 2000), 138; "Mrs. Bethune's Daytona School a 'Civilizer': Negro Teacher Tells How Her Moral and Industrial Training in Classroom and Home Prepares Pupils for True Citizenship," *New York Times*, March 5, 1916, 8; Irene R. Foote, "Report of District Public Health Nurse," in *State Board of Health of Florida Twenty-Eighth Annual Report, 1916*, 148.

29. Foote, "Report of District Public Health Nurse," 1916, 148.

30. "Florida Federation of Colored Women's Clubs Hold Interesting Session," *Freeman*, 3.

31. Fox, "Public Health Administration in Florida," 1388.

32. Terry, "Report of City Health Officer," 6.

33. Patterson, "Germs and Jim Crow," 534.

34. "The Negro and His Relation to Public Health," *Florida Health Notes* 12, no. 5 (May 1917): 98.

35. "Negro and His Relation to Public Health," 98.

36. Jennifer Ritterhouse, *Growing Up Jim Crow: How Black and White Southern Children Learned Race* (Chapel Hill: University of North Carolina Press, 2006), 11, 68.

37. Terry, "Report of City Health Officer," 6, 37.

38. Ellen Lowell-Stevens, "Report of Health Committee F.F.W.C.," in *FFWC Yearbook, 1908–1909*, 31.

39. In William A. Link, *The Paradox of Southern Progressivism, 1880–1930* (Chapel Hill: University of North Carolina Press, 1992), 187.

40. Lowell-Stevens, "Report of Health Committee," 1908–1909, 31.

41. Lowell-Stevens, "Report of Health Committee." See also Hardy and Pynchon, *Millstones and Milestones*, 121.

42. Lowell-Stevens, "Report of Health Committee," 30–35; Ellen Lowell-Stevens, "Report of Health Department Civics Committee," in *FFWC Yearbook, 1909–1910*, 43–48.

43. Hardy and Pynchon, *Millstones and Milestones*, 27.

44. Lowell-Stevens, "Report of the Health Department," 1908–1909, 34.

45. Lowell-Stevens, "Report of the Health Department Civics Committee," 1909–1910, 43.

46. Lowell-Stevens, "Report of the Health Department Civics Committee," 1909–1910, 43; Hardy and Pynchon, *Millstones and Milestones*, 23, 120.

47. Joseph Y. Porter, "Tuberculosis," in *State Board of Health of Florida Twenty-Fifth Annual Report, 1913* (Jacksonville: Drew, 1914), 18–19.

48. Joseph Y. Porter, "District Tuberculosis Nursing Plan in Florida," *Southern Medical Journal* 9, no. 8 (August 1916): 699–701.

49. Porter, "Tuberculosis," 19.

50. Ellen Lowell-Stevens, "Report from Department of Public Health, 1913–1915," *FFWC Yearbook, 1914–1915*, (Lakeland: Florida Federation of Women's Clubs, 1916), 56–57.

51. Elna C. Green, "Protecting Confederate Soldiers and Mothers' Pensions, Gender, and the Welfare State in the U.S. South: A Case Study from Florida," *Journal of Social History* 39, no. 4 (Summer 2006): 1079.

52. Seth Weitz, "Defending the Old South: The Myth of the Lost Cause and Political Immorality in Florida, 1865–68," *The Historian* 71, no. 1 (Spring 2009): 79–92; Nina Silber, *Gender and the Sectional Conflict* (Chapel Hill: University of North Carolina Press, 2008), 83, 95.

53. Green, "Protecting Confederate Soldiers and Mothers' Pensions," 1083.

54. "Florida True Friend to Ex-Confederates," *Pensacola Journal*, April 28, 1914, 8; "Florida Generous to Veterans," *Jonesboro [AR] Weekly Sun*, February 18, 1914, 7.

55. Keith S. Bannon, "'These Few Gray-Haired, Battle Scarred Veterans': Confederate Army Reunions in Georgia, 1885–95," in *The Myth of the Lost Cause and Civil War History*, ed. Gary W. Gallagher and Alan T. Nolan (Bloomington: Indiana University Press, 2000), 96.

56. In "Jacksonville, the Reunion City," *Confederate Veteran* 22, no. 4 (April 1914): 148. The journal was published in Nashville.

57. "Florida True Friend to Ex-Confederates," *Pensacola Journal*.

58. Bannon, "These Few Gray-Haired, Battle Scarred Veterans," 96.

59. Foote required five Red Cross relief stations that were supplied with nurses from Georgia, Tennessee, Louisiana, North Carolina, and of course, Florida. "Florida," *Trained Nurse and Hospital Review* (1914): 248; "New Chapters Ready for Emergencies," *American Red Cross Bulletin* 9, no. 3 (July 1914): 170.

60. "Red Cross Nurses for Reunion Relief Work," *Tampa Tribune*, April 14, 1914, 1; Jane Delano, "The Red Cross," *American Journal of Nursing* 14, no. 11 (August 1914): 966–971. For a silent movie of the 1914 Confederate reunion in Jacksonville, with "Miss Foote, the Superintendent of Nurses" pictured outside a hospital tent, see *Confederate Veterans Reunion*, 1914, video, 16:15, Mackey and Coutant Film Co., n.d., Florida Memory, https://www.floridamemory.com/items/show/232382.

61. Edna L. Foley, "Department of Visiting Nursing and Social Welfare," *American Journal of Nursing* 15, no. 12 (September 15, 1915): 1116–1117.

62. Irene R. Foote, "Results in District Tuberculosis Work," *Florida Health Notes* 11 (November 1915): 352.

63. Foote, "Report of District Public Health Nurse," 149; For all twelve nurses' reports for 1916 see *State Board of Health of Florida Twenty-Eighth Annual Report, 1916*, 141-159.

64. Karleen Gillies, "A [Long] History of the Florida Nurses Association 1909–1984," unpublished manuscript, 33–34. Author's history of nursing file.

65. Gardner, *Public Health Nursing*, 42; Hine, *Black Women in White*, 92.

66. For biographical details of the first state health nurses and a transcription and analysis of their reports see Christine Ardalan, "Florida's First State Nurses: Reporting on A Service for Health," in *Southern Women in the Progressive Era: A Reader*, ed. Giselle Roberts and Melissa Walker (Columbia: University of South Carolina Press, 2019).

67. Joseph Y. Porter, "Report of the State Health Officer," *State Board of Health of Florida Twenty-Sixth Annual Report, 1914* (Jacksonville: Drew 1915), 33–34.

68. Porter, "Report of the State Health Officer," 1914, 33.

69. W. E. Bray, "Rural Sanitation and Rural Sanitation Nurse," *Public Health Nurse Quarterly* 7, no. 1 (January 1915): 54–55.

70. Joseph Y. Porter, "General Sanitary Management," *Southern Medical Journal* 8, no. 10 (October 1915): 857.

71. Linda Vance, *May Mann Jennings, Florida's Genteel Activist* (Gainesville: University Press of Florida 1985), 91; Jessie Hamm Meyer, *Leading the Way: A Century of Service G.F.W.C. Florida Federation of Women's Clubs, 1895–1995* (Lakeland: GFWC Florida Federation of Women's Clubs, 1994), 47.

72. Porter, "General Sanitary Management."

73. Porter, "General Sanitary Management."

74. Anastatia Sims, *The Power of Femininity in the New South: Women's Organization and Politics in North Carolina, 1880–1930* (Columbia: University of South Carolina Press, 1997), 3–4; Seth Koven and Sonya Michel, "Introduction: Mother Worlds," in *Mothers of the New World: Maternalist Politics and the Origins of Welfare States* (New York: Routledge, 1993), 1–42.

75. Porter, "District Tuberculosis Nursing Plan in Florida," 701.

76. For the role of public health nurses as intermediaries see Buhler-Wilkinson, "False Dawn," 94.

77. Beardsley, *History of Neglect*, 133.

78. For typical gendered perceptions of a nurse's work and her role as the deferential member of the doctor-nurse team see John E. Boyd, "The Nurse from a Doctor's Viewpoint," *American Journal of Nursing* 13, no. 7 (April 1913): 506–507. Boyd was a surgeon and the founder of De Soto Sanitarium in Jacksonville. In this speech at the first annual convention of the State Graduate Nurses of Florida, he said, "The nurse should be the truest friend a doctor has, be his chief assistant, help him think right, . . . respect him, make him respect her, shoulder the responsibility with him."

79. Porter, "Report of the State Health Officer," 1914, 34.

80. Mary Spencer, "Report of District Public Health Nurse," 1916 143; Foote, "Report of District Public Health Nurse," 148; Susan Voorhees, "Report of District Public Health Nurse," 145; all are in *State Board of Health of Florida Twenty-Eighth Annual Report, 1916* 148–151. For doctors' lack of cooperation more generally in the South see also Beardsley, *History of Neglect*, 133; Link, *The Paradox of Southern Progressivism*, 286–287.

81. Porter, "Report of the State Health Officer," 1914, 34.

82. Bray, "Rural Sanitation and Rural Sanitation Nurse," 54.

83. Porter, "District Nursing Plan in Florida," 700.

84. Grace Whitford, "Annual Report of the Public Health Department," in *FFWC Yearbook, 1915–1916*, 78.

85. Frances Herndone was the State Board of Health's librarian. She resigned as one of the first three state health nurses to work with the Board's touring exhibits. In 1917, she was the supervisor of the Health Exhibit Train.

86. Foote, "Results in District Tuberculosis Work," 352.

87. "Reports of District Public Health Nurses," 1916, 141–159.

88. Jessie Wheeler, "Report of District Public Health Nurse," 1916, 157.

89. Rhea H. Lee, "Report of District Public Health Nurse," 1916, 155.

90. F. A. [Laura] Scott, "Report of District Public Health Nurse," 1916, 153. In her report, she uses her husband's initials, F. A.

91. Harriet Sherman, "Report of District Public Health Nurse," 1916, 142.

92. Mary Eleanor Roach, "Report of District Public Health Nurse," 1916, 150. Foote shared their concern in her "Report of District Public Health Nurse," 1916, 149.

93. Florida did not pass fence laws until the 1960s. Linda Vance, *Mary Mann Jennings: Florida's Genteel Activist* (Gainesville: University Press of Florida, 1985), 56–57.

94. "Reports of District Public Health Nurses," 1916: Spencer, 143; Foote, 149; Voorhees, 146.

95. May Mann Jennings, President FFWC, to Mrs. W. R. Cole, April 5, 1916, May Mann Jennings, Correspondence 1916, April-May, University of Florida Digital Collections, ufdc. ufl.edu.

96. In Edward H. Beardsley, *A History of Neglect Health Care for Blacks and Mill Workers in the Twentieth Century South* (Knoxville: University of Tennessee Press, 1987), 133.

97. Beardsley, *History of Neglect*, 132–133; Franklin Johnson, *The Development of State Legislation Concerning the Free Negro* (Clark, NJ: Lawbook Exchange, 2007), 25, 67, 160–161.

98. C. H. Dobbs, "District Public Health Nurses," State Board of Health of Florida Twenty-Eighth Report, 1916, 43.

99. Such fears were heightened by historical fiction like Thomas Dixon's books *The Leopard's Spots* (1902) and *The Clansman: An Historical Romance of the Ku Klux Klan* (1905) that retold Reconstruction and its aftermath to champion white supremacy and the role of the Ku Klux Klan to save white womanhood from what the books and later the play and film portray as brutal black rapists. For the rhetoric and evolution of the books and film see Gilmore, *Gender and Jim Crow*, 134–138. For the fiction of violence directed toward women see Kimberly Jensen, *Mobilizing Minerva: American Women in the First World War* (Urbana: University of Chicago Press, 2008), 22. For examples of praise in Florida of *The Leopard's Spots* play see *Pensacola Journal,* January 1, 1914, 9. A review of D. W. Griffith's film that "built spectacle on the Clansman" is "The Birth of a Nation at the Duval Theatre," *Ocala Evening Star*, November 25, 1915, 5.

100. The division of racial status was maintained in State Board of Health reports through 1936, but the difference was marked until the civil rights revolution of the 1960s. The State Board of Health annual report for 1936 was the last to list the personnel. The lone African American public health nurse was listed as Nurse Ethel Mae Jones [Kirkland], State Midwife Teacher. The white director, Ruth E. Mettinger, and eight white supervisors were called "Miss" or "Mrs." *State Board of Health of Florida Thirty-Seventh Annual Report* (Jacksonville: State Board of Health, 1937), 48.

101. Lottie Culp Gantt, "Report of District Public Health Nurse," 158–159.

102. Convention minutes, February 17, 1916, FFWC Minutes, 1914–1930, GFWC Florida Federation of Women's Clubs Headquarters, Lakeland.

103. Link, *Paradox of Southern Progressivism*, 242.

104. Link, *Paradox of Southern Progressivism*, 242.

105. Gantt, "Report of District Public Health Nurse," 158–159.

106. Fox, "Public Health Administration," 1385.

107. Foote, "Report of District Public Health Nurse," 148. For further information on Bethune's school see "Mrs. Bethune's Daytona School a 'Civilizer': Negro Teacher Tells How Her Moral and Industrial Training in Classroom and Home Prepares Pupils for True Citizenship," *New York Times*, March 5, 1916, SM8.

108. Foote, "Report of District Public Health Nurse," 148.

109. Foote, "Report of District Public Health Nurse," 148.

110. "Report of District Public Health Nurse," 1916: Foote, 148; Wheeler, 155–156; Roach, 151; Sherman, 142.

111. Since its founding in 1872, this organization had extended membership to laypersons who were interested in reforming public health initiatives. Duffy, *Sanitarians*, 130.

112. Hine, *Black Women in White*, 92.

113. Buhler-Wilkinson "False Dawn," 92.

114. Mary M. Roberts, "The Story of the Department of Nursing and Health, Teachers College, New York," *American Journal of Nursing* 21, no. 8 (May 1921): 518–524.

115. Porter, "Report of the State Health Officer," 1914, 32; Porter, "District Public Health Nursing," 42.

116. C. H. Dobbs, "District Public Health Nursing," *State Board of Health of Florida Twenty-Eighth Annual Report, 1916*, 42.

117. Joseph Y. Porter, "State Health Officer's Report," *State Board of Health of Florida Twenty-Seventh Annual Report, 1915* (Jacksonville: Drew, 1916), 18.

118. Porter, "State Health Officer's Report," 1915, 18.

119. Buhler-Wilkinson, "False Dawn," 92.

120. Boyd, "Nurse from a Doctor's Viewpoint," 506.

121. Voorhees, 145; Foote, 147–148; Scott, 153; Spencer, 143. "Report of District Public Health Nurse."

122. Porter, "District Tuberculosis Nursing Plan," 700.

123. Dr. W. H. Cox managed Catts's South Florida campaign and became the state health officer. Charles T. Frecker of Tampa, the secretary of Catts's South Florida office, became the president of the State Board of Health. They remained in office until a bitter confusion in 1919 resulted in the dismissal of both and the appointment of Joe Earman as the president of the board and Dr. Ralph Greene as the state health officer. Wayne Flynt, *Cracker Messiah: Governor Sidney J. Catts* (Baton Rouge: Louisiana State University Press, 1977), 71, 107, 111; Hardy and Pynchon, *Millstones and Milestones*, 28.

124. Sherman, "Report of District Public Health Nurse," 142.

125. Virginia Scharff, *Taking the Wheel: Women and the Coming of the Motor Age* (Albuquerque: University of New Mexico, 1991), 25.

126. Foote, "Report of District Public Health Nurse," 150.

127. Grace Whitford, "Annual Report of the Public Health Department," in *FFWC Yearbook, 1917-1918* (Lakeland: Florida Federation of Women's Clubs, 1919), 80.

128. Whitford, "Annual Report of the Public Health Committee," 80.

129. Wilson T. Sowder, "Joseph Yates Porter: The Merchants Son Who Became Florida's First State Officer," *Journal of Florida Medical Association* 54, no. 8 (August 1967): 807.

130. Harriet Sherman and Susan Voorhees became members of the American Red Cross Nursing Service. Eula Lee Paschall and Margaret Bennett (b. 1891) joined the Army Nurse Corps, and later Paschall served in Europe. The Women's Christian Temperance Union leader Laura Scott served on the executive board of the Starke Branch of the North Florida Chapter of the American Red Cross. Sherman became the state director of nurses for the Florida Anti-Tuberculosis Association in 1919. Susan Voorhees became the superintendent of nurses for Jacksonville's City Health Department. Mary Roach pursued her public health work in midwifery. And Lottie Culp Gantt pursued her outreach as a nurse for an insurance company.

131. Grace Whitford, "Report to Dr. W. H. Cox," February 13, 1919, in *State Board of Health of Florida Thirtieth Annual Report, 1918* (Jacksonville: Jacksonville Printing, 1919), 70.

132. Whitford, "Report to Dr. W. H. Cox," 70.

133. Hine, *Black Women in White*, 94.

134. In Mary F. Clark, "Of Interest to Nurses," *Journal of National Medical Association* 9, no. 1 (1917): 40.

Chapter 2. Stirring Northern Initiatives into Florida's Backwaters, 1922 to 1930

1. Laurie Jean Reid to Grace Abbott, March 7, 1923, file 4-10-4-0, box 190, record group (RG) 102, Children's Bureau (CB) Central File 1921–1924, NARA.

2. Susan L. Smith, "White Nurses, Black Midwives, and Public Health in Mississippi, 1920–1950," in *Women and Health in America*, 2nd edition, ed. Judith Walzer Leavitt (Madison: University of Wisconsin Press, 1999), 446.

3. Reid to Abbott, March 7, 1923.

4. Laurie Jean Reid, "The Sheppard-Towner Act and Its Application in Florida," *Florida Health Notes* 15, no. 8 (August 1923): 54.

5. The act was sponsored by Senator Morris Sheppard of Texas and Representative Horace Towner of Iowa; it was signed into law on November 23, 1921, by President Warren Harding.

6. Molly Ladd-Taylor, "My Work Came out of Agony and Grief: Mothers and the Making of the Sheppard-Towner Act," in *Mothers of the New World: Maternalist Politics and the Origins of Welfare States*, ed. Seth Koven and Sonya Michel (New York: Routledge, 1993), 321–323; Molly Ladd-Taylor, "'Grannies' and 'Spinsters': Midwife Education under the Sheppard-Towner Act," *Journal of Social History* 22, no. 2 (Winter 1988): 258; Muncy, *Creating a Female Dominion*, 93–123; J. Stanley Lemons, *The Woman Citizen: Social Feminism in the 1920s* (Charlottesville: University of Virginia, 1973), 153–180; Richard W. Wertz and Dorothy C. Wertz, *Lying In: A History of Childbirth in America* (New Haven, CT: Yale, 1989), 208–215; Melosh, *Physician's Hand*, 119–120.

7. Grace Abbott, "Administration of the Sheppard-Towner Act: Plans for Maternal Care," cited in the chapter "The Sheppard-Towner Act," in Bremner, *Children and Youth in America*, 2:1007.

8. The fourteen states were Alabama, Delaware, Florida, Kentucky, Michigan, Mississippi, New Jersey, North Carolina, Ohio, Pennsylvania, South Carolina, Tennessee, Utah, and Virginia. Six states planned only to conduct surveys of maternal and child health: California, Connecticut, Idaho, Maryland, Missouri, and Nevada.

9. Each year for five years, $5,000 was appropriated, with the balance of the initial $1,240,000 to be divided among the states accepting the terms of the act. Prior to Reid's arrival, Margaret Duffy of the US Public Health Service had come to Florida to prepare for the implementation of the act. Her service was discontinued on July 12, 1921. Reid, "Sheppard-Towner Act"; Laurie Jean Reid, "Report of Bureau of Child Welfare, 1921–1922," in *State Board of Health of Florida Twenty-Second Report, Biennial, 1921–1922* (Jacksonville: Record Company Printers, 1923), 91–102; W. B. Keating, "Nursing Service: Field Investigation in Child Hygiene in Florida," in *State Board of Health of Florida Twenty-Second Report, Biennial, 1921–1922*, 115.

10. Reid, "Sheppard-Towner Act."

11. Reid to Abbott, March 7, 1923.

12. Reid, "Report of Bureau of Child Welfare, 1921–1922," 94.

13. "Child Welfare Talk to the Florida State League of Women Voters," (St. Petersburg) *Evening Independent*, January 24, 1923, 7; Hardy and Pynchon, *Millstones and Milestones*, 30–31.

14. Ellen Lowell-Stevens, "Report from Department of Public Health, 1913–1915," *FFWC Yearbook, 1914–1915*, 51; Hiram Byrd, "Rough Outline of the History of the Beginning of Child Welfare Work in Florida," September 30, 1918, unfiled, GFWC Florida Federation of Women's Clubs Headquarters, Lakeland.

15. Minutes of the Florida Federation of Women's Clubs, November 19, 1918, GFWC Florida Federation of Women's Clubs Headquarters, Lakeland.

16. "Florida State Board of Health Awaits Approval for Child Welfare Program," *Miami News*, January 17, 1922; M. Josie Rogers, "Department of Public Health of the Florida Federation of Women's Clubs," *FFWC Yearbook, 1920–1921*, 94–97.

17. "Florida Rejects Aid of Sheppard-Towner Measure," *Evening Independent*, May 25, 1923, 1; "State Kills Bill for Aid of Babies," *Miami News*, May 24, 1923, 17. For the rhetoric of opposition see the chapter "The Sheppard-Towner Act" in Bremner, *Children and Youth in America*, 2:1010–1025.

18. "State Kills Bill for Aid of Babies," *Miami News*, May 24, 1923, 17.

19. Vance, *May Mann Jennings*, 108–109.

20. Laurie Jean Reid, "Public Health Nursing: A Factor in Child Welfare," *Florida Health Notes* 14, no. 8 (December 1922): 119.

21. In *American Journal of Nursing* 13, no. 7 (April 1913): 506. Boyd's speech is printed verbatim in the journal. For Boyd's place on the program for the convention in Jacksonville, January 29–31, 1913, see Gillies, *Sunshine and Breezes*, 8–9.

22. Laurie Jean Reid, "Public Health Nursing: A Factor in Child Welfare," *Florida Health Notes* 14, no. 8 (December 1922): 119.

23. The first organized federal nursing service was for the US Army in 1901, the second for the US Navy in 1908, and the third when the US Public Health Service developed its own nursing service in 1919 in response to the need for nurses to care for sick and injured World War I veterans. Ellwynne M. Vreeland, "Fifty Years of Nursing in the Federal Government Nursing Services," *American Journal of Nursing* 50, no. 10 (October 2, 1950): 626–631.

24. Smith, "White Nurses, Black Midwives," 446.

25. Muncy, *Creating a Female Dominion*, 117; Molly Ladd-Taylor, "Hull House Goes to Washington: Women and the Children's Bureau," in *Gender, Class, Race, and Reform in the Progressive Era*, ed. Noralee Frankel and Nancy S. Dye (Lexington: University of Kentucky Press, 1991), 115.

26. Laurie Jean Reid, "District Nursing under the Sheppard-Towner Act," *Florida Health Notes* 15, no. 1 (January 1923): 23.

27. "Mrs. Raymond Robbins Host to Brooksville Women at Fine Home," *Tampa Tribune*, March 13, 1923, 13.

28. Reid, "District Nursing under the Sheppard-Towner Act," 23; Laurie Jean Reid, "Square Pegs in Round Holes," *Florida Health Notes* 21, no. 10 (October 1929): 129.

29. Reid to Abbott, March 7, 1923.

30. The *New York Times* reported a sharp decrease in the number of lynchings in southern states during the first half of 1923 compared to the previous six months. Among the states, Florida had the most reported, at three; Georgia had two; Arkansas, Alabama, Louisiana, Mississippi, Missouri, and Texas had one each. "Lynchings Drop from 33 to 11 for a Six Month Period," *New York Times*, June 26, 1923, 21.

31. For Jennifer Ritterhouse's discussion of the perpetuation of mob violence and lynching in the South with particular reference to Florida see her *Growing Up Jim Crow*, 71–81. For violence and lynching in Florida see David R. Colburn, "Rosewood and America in the Early Twentieth Century," *Florida Historical Quarterly* 74, no. 2 (Fall 1997): 175–192; Maxine Jones, "The Rosewood Massacre and the Women Who Survived It," *Florida Historical Quarterly* 74, no. 2 (Fall 1997): 193–208.

32. Reid to Abbott, March 7, 1923.

33. In "State Director of Child Welfare Flays Modern Mother for Improper Training of Daughters," *St. Petersburg Times*, January 5, 1923, 1.

34. Margaret Jarman Hagood, *Mothers of the South: Portraiture of the White Tenant Farm Woman* (Charlottesville: University Press of Virginia, 1996), 7, 108–127. This is a reprint of the 1937 North Carolina Press edition.

35. Ladd-Taylor, "My Work Came out of Agony," 332. Some of Hagood's findings in her *Mothers of the South* are illuminated in mothers' letters to the Children's Bureau. An example quoted by Ladd-Taylor is that of Mrs. M. T. of Texas, who writes, "my mother taught *me nothing*, I am still paying the penalty for ignorance." In Molly Ladd-Taylor, *Raising a Baby the Government Way, 1915–1932* (New Brunswick, NJ: Rutgers, 1986), 128.

36. Lavinia Dock, "Foreign Department: The Eugenics Educational Society of England," *American Journal of Nursing* 10, no. 3 (December 1909): 187–189.

37. Constitution of the Arkansas Eugenics Association of 1930, cited in Marianne Leung, "'Better Babies': Birth Control in Arkansas during the 1930s," *Southern Women: Hidden Histories of Women of the New South*, ed. Virginia Bernhard, Betty Brandon, Elizabeth Fox-Genovese, Theda Perdue, Elizabeth H. Turner (Columbia: University of Missouri Press, 1994), 52.

38. In Laurie Jean Reid, "Child Hygiene and Public Health Nursing: 'Service,'" *Florida Health Notes* 19, no. 10 (October 1927): 131.

39. As noted in Barney, *Authorized to Heal*, 102.

40. Judith Barrett Litoff, "The Midwife as 'Necessary Evil,'" in *American Midwife Debate*,

ed. Litoff, 127–128; Debra Ann Susie, *In the Way of Our Grandmothers: A Cultural View of Twentieth-Century Midwifery in Florida* (Athens: University of Georgia Press, 1988), 8.

41. Reid to Abbott, March 7, 1923.

42. Reid to Abbott, March 7, 1923; Laurie Jean Reid, "Manual of Instruction for Midwives," 1924, file 19, carton 2, series 904, Midwife Program File, Florida State Archives, Tallahassee.

43. Wertz and Wertz, *Lying In*, 213–215; Beardsley, *History of Neglect*, 39–41; Ladd-Taylor, "My Work Came out of Agony," 321–322.

44. Smith, "White Nurses, Black Midwives," 444–458.

45. Laurie Jean Reid, "Report of the Bureau of Child Welfare, Florida State Board of Health 1921–22," in *State Board of Health of Florida Thirty-Second Report Biennial, 1921–1922* (Jacksonville: State Board of Health), 94.

46. Laurie Jean Reid, "Report to Grace Abbott," March 1924, "Reports to Grace Abbott," January–December 1924, file 11-11-1, box 245, RG 102, CB Central File, 1921–1924, NARA.

47. Laurie Jean Reid, "All in the Day's Work," *Florida Health Notes* 18, no. 1 (January 1926): 178–179.

48. Laurie Jean Reid, "Infant Welfare Clinics," *Florida Health Notes* 15, no. 4 (January 1923): 61. Further details about the clinics are in Laurie Jean Reid, "Report to Grace Abbott," February 1924, file 11-11-1, box 245, RG 102, CB Central File, 1921–1924, NARA.

49. Laurie Jean Reid to Grace Abbott, letter, September 7, 1925, file 11-11-1, box 325, RG 102, CB Central File, 1925–1928, NARA.

50. Goggans, "Wonderful Years."

51. Ladd-Taylor, "My Work Came out of Agony," 333.

52. Laurie Jean Reid, "Sheppard-Towner Act and Its Application in Florida," GFWC *Florida Federation of Women's Clubs Yearbook, 1927–1928*, 144–145.

53. A summary of "Accomplishments under the Maternity and Infancy Act" is in "Florida," Report to the Children's Bureau, unsigned [Laurie Jean Reid], 1928, p. 2, file 11-0 box 318, RG 102, CB Central File, 1925–1928, NARA.

54. The nurses' specific activities toward birth registration are found in Laurie Jean Reid, "Reports to Children's Bureau," March, April, and October 1924. For "Admission of States to Death and Birth Registration Areas" see Bremner, *Children and Youth in America*, 965.

55. "Florida," report for the Children's Bureau, unsigned [Laurie Jean Reid], September 7, 1926, file 11-0, box 318, RG 102, CB Central File, 1925–1928, NARA.

56. Melosh, *Physician's Hand*, 128–129.

57. "Florida," report for the Children's Bureau, September 7, 1926, p. 3.

58. Anne O'Hare McCormick, "Adventuring in Our Tropical Empire," *New York Times*, March 15, 1925, 2; "Camp Sanitation Worries Florida," *Berkeley Daily Gazette*, January 2, 1926, 13.

59. Reid to Abbott, letter, September 7, 1925. For a succinct account of the tourist camps see Tebeau, *History of Florida*, 383–386.

60. Laurie Jean Reid, "Report of Activities of the Division of Maternal and Infant Hygiene, Bureau of Child Welfare and Public Health Nursing, Florida State Board of Health for the Month of August," 1925, file 11-11-1, box 325, CB Central File, 1925–1928, NARA.

61. Reid, "Child Hygiene and Public Health Nursing: 'Service,'" 132.

62. Reid to Abbott, letter, September 7, 1925; Laurie Jean Reid, "All in the Day's Work," *Florida Health Notes* 18, no. 1 (January 1926): 178–179.

63. Reid to Abbott, letter, September 7, 1925; Laurie Jean Reid, "Report to the Children's Bureau," August 1925, file 11-11-1, box 325, RG 102, CB Central File, 1925–1928, NARA.

64. Reid to Abbott, letter, September 7, 1925.

65. Laurie Jean Reid, "Report to Grace Abbott," May 1924. For the number of nurses per year see the annual reports of 1924–1930 in *Decade in Public Health*, 52–63.

66. Laurie Jean Reid, "Report to the State Board of Health," in *Decade in Public Health*, 55. The eight counties were Volusia, Brevard, Putnam, Marion, Alachua, Escambia, St. Lucie, and Palm Beach.

67. H. Hanson, "Decade in Public Health," 4. In her early reports to the Children's Bureau, Reid used the title of director, Bureau of Child Welfare and Public Health Nursing.

68. M. Josie Rogers, "Department of Public Welfare Report of Chairman Division of Child Welfare, *FFWC Yearbook, 1924–1926*, 96.

69. Reid, "Report to Grace Abbott," February 1924.

70. Pierce was a phosphate mining town owned and operated by the American Agricultural Chemical Company. It was one of many places in Polk County where there were few roads or automobiles and residents were dependent upon company-owned housing, utilities, and health care.

71. Laurie Jean Reid, "Report to Grace Abbott," September 1924, file 11-11-1, box 245, CB Central File, 1921–1924, NARA.

72. Gardner, *Public Health Nursing*, 204.

73. Laurie Jean Reid, "A Trip with a Movie Truck," *Florida Health Notes* 16, no. 6 (June 1924): 86–89.

74. In 1923 the American Child Health Association designated May 1 as Child Health Day. In 1928 Congress sanctioned the date, and President Calvin Coolidge proclaimed May 1 as National Child Health Day. Laurie Jean Reid, "The First of May Is Every Child's Day," *Florida Health Notes* 19, no. 4 (April 1927): 60–63.

75. Smith, *Sick and Tired*, 36, 50.

76. B. L. Arms, "A Pressing Need in Florida" *Florida Health Notes* 17, no. 12 (December 1925): 155.

77. In Smith, *Sick and Tired*, 36.

78. Raymond C. Turck, "Administration: National Negro Health Week," *Florida Health Notes* 17, no. 3 (March 1925): 30.

79. Laurie Jean Reid, "Report to Grace Abbott," April 1925, file 11-11-1, box 325, CB Central File, 1925–1928, NARA.

80. "Classes in Nursing for Negro Women Are Opened by Red Cross," *Tampa Tribune*, March 22, 1923, 20; "Home Hygiene Classes Are Wanted by Many," *Tampa Tribune*, October 3, 1914, 11.

81. "Negro Department," *Tampa Tribune*, March 7, 1924, 17.

82. "State Worker Arrives Here," *St. Petersburg Times*, July 21, 1923, 7.

83. Minutes, NACGN Convention, 1925, NACGN Records. Bertha E. Deen was the superintendent of Brewster Hospital and Training School for Nurses from 1919 to 1929. Sessions, *Charge to Keep*, 30.

84. Minutes, NAGCN convention, 1925.

85. Officials of the State Board of Health were Calvin T. Young, president, from Plant City;

Charles H. Mann, Jacksonville, and F. Clifton Moor, Tallahassee. John W. Martin, whom Mettinger referenced, served as governor of Florida from January 6, 1925, to January 8, 1929. Dr. B. L. Arms replaced Dr. Turck for a four-year term as the state health officer in 1925. William J. Bigler, "Public Health in Florida—Yesteryear," *Florida's Journal of Public Health* 1, no. 3 (May 1989): 7.

86. Laurie Jean Reid, "Report to Grace Abbott," May 1926, file 11-11-8, box 325, RG 102, CB Central File, 1925–1928, NARA.

87. Charlotte Heilman, employed by the National Red Cross Nursing Service, was its nursing field representative for Florida. She conducted monthly visits to report on the nursing activities furnished by the state's Red Cross chapters. She noted that St. Augustine's Red Cross chapter engaged Bonner to conduct a home hygiene program in the industrial school as well as other public health work. Heilman, "Nursing Field Representative Report," August 1926, file 159.1, box 255, RG 200, American National Red Cross Records (hereafter ANRC Records).

88. Charlotte Heilman, "Efficiency Report," May 1, 1926, Mettinger, Ruth Esther, Historical Nurse files, box 62, RG 200, ANRC Records.

89. Ida Malinde Havey, "Efficiency Report for Nursing Field Representative," June 25, 1928, Mettinger file, ANRC Records. Havey was an assistant director of the Red Cross Public Health Nursing Service. Public health nursing had become a growing field within the National Red Cross Nursing Service.

90. Ruth Mettinger to Elizabeth C. Fox, November 12, 1928, Mettinger file, ANRC Records.

91. Mettinger to Fox, November 12, 1928.

92. The Red Cross Public Health Nursing Service was distinct from the Red Cross Nursing Service, which was formed earlier as a corps of nurses ready for disaster relief work.

93. "Report of Public Health Nursing Services in Area Stations," Florida Hurricane, 9/18/1926, box 750, Central File 200, 1917–1934, ANRC Records. "Health Activities West Indian Hurricane," Hurricane: 9/13/28, box 753, RG 200, 1917–1934, ANRC Records. See William M. Straight, "Killer 'Canes and Medical Care," *Journal of the Florida Medical Association* 62, no. 8 (August 1975): 35–42. The 1928 hurricane of September 16 was also known as the San Felipe, Okeechobee, and Florida Everglades hurricane.

94. Clara D. Noyes, "Department of Red Cross Nursing: Florida Hurricane Disaster," *American Journal of Nursing* 26, no. 11 (November 1926): 884; Laurie Jean Reid to Elizabeth G. Fox, American Red Cross Director of Nursing, "Health Activities West Indian Hurricane Florida Area," September 30, 1928, box 753, RG 200, 1917–1934, ANRC Records.

95. Laurie Jean Reid, "The Daily Task," *Florida Health Notes* 20, no. 10–11 (October–November 1928): 145–146.

96. Laurie Jean Reid to Grace Abbott, September 18, 1926, file 11-11-1, box 325, RG 102, CB Central File, 1925–1928, NARA.

97. Steven Noll addresses the consequences of Reid's endorsement to "weed out weaklings" in "'A Far Greater Menace': Feebleminded Females in the South," in *Hidden Histories of Women in the New South*, ed. Virginia Bernhard (Columbia: University of Missouri Press, 1994), 32.

98. Lavinia Dock, "Foreign Department: The Eugenics Educational Society of England," *American Journal of Nursing* 10, no. 3 (December 1909): 187.

99. A policy based on eugenics led to forced sterilization of poor women and experimentation without patient consent. Such practices of medical abuses especially of African Ameri-

cans followed the pattern of abuses African Americans had endured during slavery. Sharla M. Fett, *Working Cures: Healing, Health, and Power on Southern Slave Plantations* (Chapel Hill: University of North Carolina Press, 2002), 2.

100. John Hurty, "Practical Eugenics," *American Journal of Nursing* 12, no. 5 (February 1912): 453.

101. Reid, "Public Health Nursing: A Factor in Child Welfare," 119.

102. Reid, "Child Hygiene and Public Health Nursing: 'Service,'" 132.

103. I. Malinde Havey, "Report of Visit to Florida," November 2, 1927, box 564, Florida Public Health folder, RG 2, 1917–1934, ANRC Records.

104. Reid, "Child Hygiene and Public Health Nursing: Service," 131.

105. Havey, "Report of Visit to Florida," November 2, 1927.

106. Havey, "Report of Visit to Florida," November 2, 1927.

107. Bertyne Anderson to Miss [Clara] Noyes, November 16, 1926, box 3, Historical Nurse files, ANRC Records; Gillies, *History of the Florida Nurses Association,* 103.

108. Havey, "Report of Visit to Florida," November 2, 1927.

109. Ruth E. Mettinger to Malinde Havey December 27, 1931, Florida Public Health file, box 564, RG 200, 1917–1934, ANRC Records.

110. Lemons, *Woman Citizen,* 172–173; Ladd-Taylor, "My Work Came out of Agony," 337.

111. Reid, "Sheppard-Towner Act and Its Application in Florida," *Federation of Women's Clubs Yearbook,* 144–146. President Calvin Coolidge signed the two-year extension into law on January 22, 1927.

112. Laurie Jean Reid, "What We Have Accomplished," *Florida Health Notes* 21, no. 8 (August 1929): 98.

113. On the continuing dire need for public health nurses in rural areas see H. Hanson, "Decade in Public Health," 10; "Expiration and Achievements of the Maternity and Infancy Act, 1929," *United States Children's Bureau, Eighteenth Annual Report,* in Bremner, *Children and Youth in America,* 1008–1009.

114. Smith, "White Nurses, Black Midwives," 446.

115. Laurie Jean Reid, "Principles of School Nursing," *Florida Health Notes* 21, no. 1 (January 1929): 17.

Chapter 3. Linking to Public Health Nursing the Red Cross Way, 1919 to 1930

1. Rosa L. Brown, "An Experiment That Won Permanency," *Red Cross Courier* 12, no. 6 (December 1932): 185.

2. Rosa L. Brown, "Rural Nursing in Palm Beach County," *National News Bulletin* (Official Organ of the NACGN) 7, no. 5 (February–March 1935), n.p., folder 1, reel 1, box 3, NACGN Records.

3. Brown, "Rural Nursing in Palm Beach County."

4. Frances Smith Dean, "Rosa L. Brown's Contribution to Her Own Race," *American Journal of Nursing* 31, no. 7 (July 1931): 841–842.

5. For other publications see for example, Rosa L. Brown, "A Negro Nurse in the 'Glades," *Opportunity Journal of Negro Life* 15, no. 11 (November 1937): 336–338, folder 8, box 2, reel 2, NACGN Records.

6. Dean, "Rosa L. Brown's Contributions," 841-842. For Brown's discussion of her own work see also Rosa L. Brown, "Public Health Nurse and Field in Which She Works in Palm Beach County," in *Annual Report to the Red Cross, 1934*, box 1, Red Cross file, Palm Beach Historical Society.

7. Brown, "Rural Nursing in Palm Beach County." Such scare tactics are well documented in S. Smith, *Sick and Tired*, 39–41.

8. In S. Smith, *Sick and Tired*, 41.

9. Brown, "Rural Nursing in Palm Beach County."

10. Brown, "Rural Nursing in Palm Beach County."

11. Brown, "Negro Nurse in the 'Glades," 338.

12. Brown, "Experiment That Won Permanency."

13. In the South there were fifteen organizations that addressed health in black communities including the American Red Cross and the National Tuberculosis Association. Smith, *Sick and Tired*, 44.

14. In Dean, "Rosa L. Brown's Contributions," 841–842.

15. In Dean "Rosa L. Brown's Contributions," 842.

16. Lowell-Stevens, "Report of Health Committee F.F.W.C." *FFWC Yearbook, 1909–1910*.

17. Brown, "Experiment That Won Permanency"; Dean, "Rosa L. Brown's Contribution."

18. Brown, "Rural Nursing in Palm Beach County."

19. Brown, "Negro Nurse in the 'Glades."

20. Brown, "Experiment That Won Permanency."

21. Brown, "Experiment That Won Permanency."

22. Dock, *History of American Red Cross Nursing*, 1.

23. Hine, *Black Women in White*, 106.

24. Adah B. Thoms, *Pathfinders: A History of Progress of Colored Graduate Nurses* (New York: Garland, 1985), 155–159.

25. Brown, "Negro Nurse in the 'Glades."

26. In Annie M. Brainard, *The Evolution of Public Health Nursing* (Philadelphia: Saunders, 1922), 302.

27. Julia E. Irwin, "Nurses without Borders: History of Nursing as U.S. International History," *Nursing History Review* 19 (2011): 94.

28. Clara D. Noyes, "The Red Cross," *American Journal of Nursing* 20, no. 2 (November 1919): 134–138.

29. On the delay in accepting African American nurses into the American Red Cross Nursing Service see "The Colored Nurses Were Not Accepted in the Red Cross Nursing Association until the Eleventh Hour," in "Colored Nurses Hold Convention," in "Of Interest to Nurses," *Journal of the National Medical Association* 12, no. 1 (January–March 1920): 49.

30. Thoms, *Pathfinders*, 155.

31. Minutes, NACGN Convention, August 22, 1917, NACGN Records. For an overall account of the Red Cross recruitment of white nurses in the war see Dock, "The European War," in *History of American Red Cross Nursing*, 387–393.

32. Delano to Thoms, in *Pathfinders*, 158–159.

33. Dora E. Thompson, Superintendent, Army Nurse Corps, to Jane A. Delano, November 14, 1918, Negro Personnel, 1917–1934, file 300.1, box 392, RG 200, ANRC Records.

34. In Minutes, NACGN Convention, 1918.

35. Mary T. Sarnecky, *A History of the U.S. Army Nurse Corps* (Philadelphia: University of Pennsylvania Press, 1999), 128.

36. "List of Red Cross Negro Nurse Enrollment, 1918 to 1949," file 300.1, box 392, RG 200, ANRC Records.

37. Dock, *History of American Red Cross Nursing*, 358; Jean Waldman Shulman, "History of the American Red Cross Badge," *American Red Cross Nursing Matters Past and Present* 13 (Winter 2014): 5–7.

38. Jane A. Delano to Division Directors, June 10, 1918, American Red Cross Nursing Service Enrollment Records, 1909–2000, file 320.2, box 392, RG 200, ANRC Records.

39. Susan Barks, number 49A, was admitted on September 4, 1918, and Mary Allen, 103A, on October 24, 1919. List of Red Cross Nurse Enrollment, 1918–1949, Nurse Enrollment Records, file 320.2, box 392, RG 200, ANRC Records. On Brown's official title see Shulman, "Introducing Rosa L. Brown."

40. In 1919 the nurses' request for military rank did not pass congressional approval. In 1920 a modified law conferring "relative rank" secured a "pseudo" officer status on nurses but did not offer a corresponding salary or official position in the hierarchy. Passage of the Army-Navy Nurses Act of 1947 and the Women's Armed Services Integration Act of 1948 ensured that military nurses would receive commissions, pay, and benefits commensurate with their rank. Jensen, *Mobilizing Minerva*, 143.

41. Ada M. Whyte to Elizabeth Fox, acting director, Red Cross Bureau of Public Health Nursing, March 24, 1919, Whyte, Ada Mabel, at " U.S., American Red Cross Nurse Files, 1916–1959," Ancestry.com and NARA, https://www.ancestry.com/search/collections/arcnursefileswwi/.

42. For the start of Whyte's work as the director of nursing services for the Florida Tuberculosis Association see "Health Clinic [Will] Be Held Here Friday," *Pensacola Journal*, February 22, 1922, 9; "Health Clinics to Be Opened Here First of February," *Palatka Daily News*, January 25, 1922, 4; "Tuberculosis Clinic Will Be Held in Punta Gorda," *Punta Gorda Herald*, April 28, 1922, 2.

43. Portia B. Kernodle, *The Red Cross Nurse in Action* (New York: Harper, 1949), 3.

44. Link, *Paradox of Southern Progressivism*, 220–221.

45. Fannie F. Clement, "Courage and a Deep Sense of Service in a Difficult, Untouched Field," *Red Cross Courier* 12, no. 6 (December 1932): 177–178.

46. Jane Van de Vrede was born in Wisconsin and graduated in 1908 from the Milwaukee County Hospital Training School for Nurses. She enrolled in the Red Cross in 1912. Van de Vrede, Jane, Historical Nurse files, box 92, ANRC Records.

47. Jane Van de Vrede, "Southern Division Report on the Bureau of Public Health Nursing, July 1, 1919 to January 1, 1920," Florida Public Health file, 1917–1934, box 564, RG 200, ANRC Records.

48. Joe Earman, a supporter of Governor Sidney Catts, took over as president of the State Board of Health in 1919. Flynt, *Cracker Messiah*, 203.

49. Link, *Paradox of Southern Progressivism*, xii.

50. "Our Red Cross Home Workers Nurse Service," *Tropical Sun*, August 22, 1919, 1.

51. Joe Earman, "Some Recent Correspondence," *Palm Beach Post*, September 10, 1919, 2.

52. "Red Cross Co-Operates with Board of Health," *Palm Beach Post*, February 9, 1920, 1.

53. Earman, "Some Recent Correspondence," 2.

54. Link, *Paradox of Southern Progressivism*, 187.

55. Summary of her career prior to 1933, unsigned, n.d., Van de Vrede, Jane, box 92, Historical Nurse files, ANRC Records.

56. Ruth Adamson, "November 1919, Narrative Report of Public Health Nursing Activities in Tennessee and Florida," box 564, Florida Public Health files, 1917–1934, RG 200, ANRC Records.

57. Adamson, "November 1919."

58. Jane Van de Vrede, in "The Need for Negro Public Health Nurses and the Provision Being Made for It," *Journal of the National Medical Association* 13, no. 1 (1921): 55–57.

59. Brown was the chairwoman of the membership committee. Her survey is in Minutes, NACGN Convention, August 16, 1921, NACGN Records.

60. Initially Van de Vrede asked for a conference to discuss the service of public health nursing in the South with Sylvia Thomas, the correspondence secretary. "Nurses Section," *Journal of the National Medical Association* 13, no. 1 (1921): 59.

61. Van de Vrede, "Need for Negro Public Health Nurses."

62. Thoms, "The Development of Colored Health Centers," in *Pathfinders*, 169–195; minutes, NACGN convention, August 20, 1920, NACGN Records.

63. In Thoms, *Pathfinders*, 193.

64. Thoms, *Pathfinders,* 191–194.

65. Taylor was a graduate of the Hampton School for Nurses in Virginia. Thoms, *Pathfinders*, 30; "Nurse Notes," *Journal of the National Medical Association* 13, no. 3 (1921): 217.

66. In 1920 the four chapters were in Apalachicola, Pensacola, Tampa, and West Palm Beach. By 1930, fifteen chapters had established public health nursing services, and eighteen had classes in home hygiene and care of the sick. Florida, 1917–1934, file 159.1, box 264, RG 200, ANRC Records.

67. Ely's return to her alma mater is noted in the US Census of 1920. For other biographical detail see Kim Curry, "Pioneer in Florida Public Health Nursing: The Work of Joyce Ely, RN," *Florida Public Health Review* 2 (2005): 17–22.

68. "Many Negro Women in Home Hygiene Classes," *Tampa Tribune*, May 22, 1923, 5.

69. In "Classes in Nursing for Negro Women Are Opened by Red Cross," *Tampa Tribune*, March 22, 1923, 20.

70. "New Red Cross Soon to Receive Certificates," *Tampa Tribune*, April 22, 1923, 6.

71. "Tampa Chapter, Red Cross: Negro Department," *Tampa Tribune*, May 7, 1924, 17.

72. Jane Van de Vrede, "Fiscal Year Report," July 30, 1924, Florida Public Health file, 1917–1934, box 564, RG 200, ANRC Records.

73. Curry, "Pioneer in Florida Public Health Nursing."

74. Meghan H. Martinez, "Racial Violence and Competing Memory in Taylor County, Florida, 1922," master's thesis, Florida State University, 2008.

75. Van de Vrede, "Fiscal Year Report," July 30, 1924.

76. Minutes, NACGN convention, 1925, Jacksonville, NACGN Records.

77. Charlotte M. Heilman, "Monthly Reports," April 1926–August 1927, Florida Nursing file, box 255, RG 200, ANRC; Muncy, *Creating a Female Dominion*, 110.

78. Dock, *History of American Red Cross Nursing*, 17–18.

79. Clara D. Noyes, "Department of Red Cross Nursing: Florida Hurricane Disaster," *America Journal of Nursing* 26, no. 11 (November 1926): 884.

80. Such efficient relief work that was first envisioned by Jane Delano had finally come to fruition. Jane A. Delano, "The Red Cross," *American Journal of Nursing* 12, no. 6 (March 1912): 486. For a summary of the process see Patrick E. Gilbo, *American Red Cross: The First Century* (New York: Harper and Row, 1981), 29–30. For relief work in Florida's Hurricanes of 1926 and 1928 see Florida Hurricane Health Activities 9/18/26, Central File, box 730, RG 200, ANRC (hereafter cited as Florida Hurricane); "Health Activities West Indian Hurricane," Florida Area, 9/13/28, Central File, 1917–1934, box 753, RG 200, ANRC Records (hereafter cited as Health Activities West Indian Hurricane); Jay Barnes, *Florida's Hurricane History* (Chapel Hill: University of North Carolina Press, 2007), 111–126; William M. Straight, "Killer 'Canes and Medical Care," *Journal of Florida Medical Association* 62, no. 8 (August 1975): 35–42.

81. Bertyne C. Anderson to Miss [Clara] Noyes, July 6, 1918, Historical Nurse files, box 3, ANRC Records.

82. Gillies, "History of the Florida Nurses Association," 103; Laurie Jean Reid, "The Public Health Nurse in Disaster Work," *Florida Health Notes* 18, no. 11 (November 1926): 161.

83. "The Florida Hurricane, September 18, 1926, Official Report of the Relief Activities," American National Red Cross, courtesy of American Red Cross, Washington, DC; Straight, "Killer 'Canes and Medical Care."

84. Noyes, "Department of Red Cross Nursing," 881.

85. Olive Chapman, "First Narrative Report from the Nursing Service," October 16, 1926, Florida Hurricane.

86. Chapman recorded 341 nurses and 100 volunteers, including married Red Cross nurses. Chapman, "First Narrative Report," Florida Hurricane.

87. Mary G. Fraser, "Miami, Florida," n.d., Florida Hurricane; Chapman, "First Narrative Report."

88. Fraser, "Miami, Florida."

89. Reid, "Field Report of Laurie Jean Reid 9/23/26"; Reid, "Mrs. Reid, Fort Lauderdale, Sept. 24, 1926"; Fraser, "Miami, Florida."

90. Reid, "Public Health Nurse in Disaster Work."

91. Reid, "Field Report of Laurie Jean Reid 9/23/26."

92. In Laurie Jean Reid, "Report of Public Health Nursing Services in Area Station North-Ward of Arch Creek to West Palm Beach, including Glades," n.d., Florida Hurricane.

93. In Reid, "Report of Public Health Nursing Services in Area Station."

94. In Reid, "Report of Public Health Nursing Services in Area Station."

95. Reid, "Report of Public Health Nursing Services in Area Station."

96. Reid, "Report of Public Health Nursing Services in Area Station."

97. Redden's reasoning regarding the employment of doctors is recorded in his report to Henry M. Baker, the overall director of disaster relief: "It was my own opinion after four careful surveys of all areas that no such emergency existed but because it was necessary to protect ourselves and the public . . . [he] agreed to send for a sufficient number of doctors to cover the situation. This resulted in 26 doctors reporting." William R. Redden, "Florida Hurricane Sept. 18, 1926," Florida Hurricane.

98. Melinda Havey, the associate director of Red Cross Public Health Nursing, went to direct nursing in Puerto Rico. Report from "Disaster Preparedness," July 1, 1928–June 30, 1929," ANRC Records.

99. Laurie Jean Reid, "The Daily Tasks," *Florida Health Notes* 20, no. 10–11 (October–November 1928): 145.

100. Straight, "Killer 'Canes and Medical Care"; Eliot Kleinberg, *Black Cloud: The Great Florida Hurricane of 1928* (New York: Carroll and Graf, 2003); Ralph Wallace, "Death in the Everglades," *Readers Digest*, October 1945, 34–37.

101. Stuart G. Thompson, the director Florida's Bureau of Vital Statistics, put the figure at 1,833, with Belle Glade suffering the highest loss, at 611. South Bay lost 247; Pahokee, 153; Miami Locks, 99; Chosen, 23. Deaths in other places varied from 1 to 11. Thompson, "Mortality from Storm," *Florida Health Notes* (October–November 1928), 155.

102. Straight, Barnes, and Kleinberg note higher estimations of deaths. Straight's estimate was slightly higher at 1,836. Kleinberg reports the number at 2,500 and Barnes as high as 3,500. Straight, "Killer 'Canes and Medical Care," 39; Kleinberg, *Black Cloud*, xiv; Barnes, *Florida's Hurricane History*, 127.

103. Stuart B. Schwartz, "Hurricanes and the Shaping of Circum-Caribbean Societies," *Florida Historical Quarterly* 83, no. 4 (Spring 2005): 407.

104. Relief workers had trouble identifying the drowned bodies. Most could not be identified due to the rapid decomposition of the bodies. See Kleinberg's chapter "The Interior" in *Black Cloud*, 139–156.

105. For the way memory affects oral histories, see Michael Frisch, "The Voice of the Past," in *The Oral History Reader*, ed. Robert Perks and Alistair Thomson (London: Routledge, 1998), 34. See also Jacqueline Dowd Hall, "Documenting Diversity: The Southern Experience," *Oral History Review* 4 (1976): 19–28.

106. Graves's notes, "In Sept 19—" and "In Sept 1933," Midwifery folder, W. M. Straight Medical Collection, Florida International University Special Collections.

107. Graves, "In Sept 19—." Graves was assigned to Pahokee, Canal Point, and adjacent points. Laurie Jean Reid and Elizabeth G. Fox, "Conference between Miss Fox and Mrs. L. J. Reid, September 30, 1928," Health Activities West Indian Hurricane.

108. Graves, "In Sept 1933."

109. Elizabeth Fox to Clara Noyes, October 2, 1928, Health Activities West Indian Hurricane.

110. In Addition to Graves's assignment, Reid assigned Niblock to the territory south of West Palm Beach including Fort Lauderdale and McLaughlin to all the territory north of West Palm Beach including Stuart. Reid and Fox, "Conference between Miss Fox and Mrs. L. J. Reid, September 30, 1928."

111. Elizabeth Fox to Clara Noyes, October 2, 1928, Health Activities West Indian Hurricane.

112. Elizabeth Fox, "Progress Report—Nursing Service October 5, 1928," Health Activities West Indian Hurricane.

113. In Kleinberg, *Black Cloud*, 166-167.

114. The accounting was arranged through the Red Cross Medical Relief Policy. Elizabeth G. Fox, "Progress Report—Nursing Service October 5, 1928."

115. Ruth Mettinger, "Final Report of Nursing Services December 22, 1928," Health Activities West Indian Hurricane.

116. Mettinger, "Final Report of Nursing Services December 22, 1928."

117. Elizabeth G. Fox to Ruth Mettinger, November 12, 1928, Health Activities West Indian Hurricane.

118. Clara D. Noyes, "Widespread Disasters," *American Journal of Nursing* 26, no. 12 (December 1926): 970.

119. Brown, "Experiment That Won Permanency," 185.

120. Duffy, *Sanitarians*, 249.

Chapter 4. Reaching Out to Midwives and Country People, 1930 to 1947

1. In a handwritten note dated October 1954 Jule O. Graves wrote, "I woke up early something after 4.00 a.m. It seemed a real message to me to work on my book without delay." This, her other handwritten notes, and her unpublished manuscript, "Midwife Program in Florida," courtesy of William M. Straight, who obtained them from the Library of the State Board of Health in Jacksonville in 1980 and shared them with the author. They are now archived in the Midwifery file of the Straight Collection. Graves's photographs, many with handwritten notes, and her other handwritten and typed documents with some that duplicate those in the Straight Collection are in Midwife Program files, 1924–1975, series 904, carton 1, file folder 5, Florida State Archives, Tallahassee. See also Jule O. Graves, "The Midwife Program in Florida," *Public Health Nursing* 31 (October 1939): 527–531.

2. Accompanying note to the photograph *African American Midwife in Broward County*, ca. 1933, black-and-white photoprint, 5 × 3 inches, State Archives of Florida, Florida Memory, https://www.floridamemory.com/items/show/44714.

3. Ladd-Taylor, "'Grannies' and 'Spinsters,'" 264.

4. Laurie Jean Reid to Grace Abbott, March 7, 1923, file 4-10-4-0, box 190, RG 102, CB Central File, 1921–1924, NARA.

5. Graves, "Midwife Program in Florida," unpublished manuscript, 5.

6. Ethel J. Kirkland, "Memory Jewels of Jule O. Graves," October 1973, 6, series 4, box 15, ACNM Records. Kirkland wrote this tribute "from the point of view of some of her friends" in response to the Florida Public Health Association decision to honor Graves with a plaque in the association's Hall of Memory as one of the "outstanding pioneers involved in public health in the past." Kirkland, introduction to "Memory Jewels," n.p.

7. Kirkland, "Memory Jewels," 11. See also Goggans, "Wonderful Years."

8. Fred L. Adair, "Prenatal and Maternal Care," *White House Conference 1930: Address and Abstracts of Committee Reports* (New York: Century, 1931), 81–83; see also Ladd-Taylor, *Raising a Baby the Government Way*, 179.

9. H. L. Harrell Sr., "Fifty Years of Medical Practice," *Journal of Florida Medical Association* 71, no. 7 (July 1984): 475.

10. Grace Higgs, interview by the author, October 22, 1997, Miami.

11. George Simpson, "Reflections through a Mirror—Darkly: The History of Medical Care in Miami's Black Community," part 1, *Miami Medicine*, January 1995, 16.

12. Verneka Silva, interview by the author, September 15, 1995, Miami. Other oral history interviews conducted by the author in Miami are those of Thelma Anderson Gibson, October 23, 1995; Idella Hogan, September 18, 1995; and Gracie Wychie, December 9, 1997.

13. Jule Graves, handwritten note, untitled, first line "A few people. Felt eyes staring at me," n.d., Midwifery file, Straight Collection.

14. Ritterhouse, *Growing Up Jim Crow*, 25–28, 41, 46.

15. Wilson T. Sowder, MD MPH, to William M. Straight, MD, December 1, 1980, Midwifery file, Straight Collection. Sowder began working on a venereal disease control program in 1940. Five years later he became the state health officer and served until 1966. Hardy and Pynchon, *Millstones and Milestones*, 53.

16. Susan "Sue" Mary Rose Floyd Graves to Mary Faith Floyd McAdoo, Atkinson-Floyd Papers, series 2, box 1, folder 1.03, Special Collections, Kennesaw State University, GA; Rose Floyd, "Muamer's Cure for Cowardice," *Cosmopolitan Monthly Illustrated Magazine*, September 1886–February 1887, 229–232.

17. In Sims, *Power of Femininity*, 127.

18. Kirkland, "Memory Jewels," 9.

19. Virginia Bernhard, *Southern Women Histories and Identities* (Columbia: University of Missouri Press, 1992), 3; Sims, *Power of Femininity*, 3–5; Joan Marie Johnson, *Southern Ladies, New Women: Race, Religion and Clubwomen in South Carolina, 1890-1930* (Gainesville: University Press of Florida, 2005), 17–19.

20. Graves, back of the photograph *Portrait of Male Midwife Uncle Ab*, ca. 1933, black-and-white photoprint, 5 × 3 inches, State Archives of Florida, Florida Memory, https://www.floridamemory.com/items/show/44606.

21. Jule Graves, "Data and Old Superstitions Gathered by the State Midwife Consultant, Florida State Board of Health," n.d., Midwifery file, Straight Collection.

22. Jule Graves, "Data and Old Superstitions."

23. William M. Straight, "Throw Downs, Fixin, Rooting, and Hexing," *Journal of Florida Medical Association* 70, no. 8 (August 1983): 635–641.

24. Jule Graves, "Kunjer," n.d., Midwifery file, Straight Collection.

25. In the early twentieth century the medical management of preeclampsia-eclampsia rested on two diverse approaches. One was conservative management that included bed rest, sedation, and morphine; the other involved the administration of intravenous magnesium sulfate, a treatment that remains in use today. As the treatment with magnesium sulfate did not evolve into the mainstream until after 1925, when it was first used at a Los Angeles Hospital, it is unlikely the treatment was available for the "conjured" woman even if Graves could facilitate her hasty removal to a hospital. For succinct historical perspectives on preeclampsia-eclampsia see Mandy J. Bell, "A Historical Overview of Preeclampsia-Eclampsia," *Journal of Obstetrics, Gynecology Neonatal Nursing* 39, no. 5 (September 2010): 510–518; Marshall D. Lindheimer, "The Historical Perspective of Preeclampsia and Eclampsia as Seen by a Nephrologist," *Clinical Review* (January–February 2013): 24–34.

26. Graves, "Data and Old Superstitions."

27. Sharla M. Fett, *Working Cures: Healing, Health, and Power on Southern Slave Plantations* (Chapel Hill: University of North Carolina Press, 2002), 42.

28. By 1900 gonococcal blindness was preventable by dropping 1 percent silver nitrate into the eye immediately after birth. Wertz and Wertz, *Lying In*, 140.

29. Kirkland, "Memory Jewels," 13.

30. Walter Blair, "Traditions in Southern Humor," *American Quarterly* 5, no. 2 (Summer 1952): 132–142.

31. Blair, "Traditions in Southern Humor," 132.

32. Jule O. Graves, "Divine Guidance," n.d., Midwifery file, Straight Collection.

33. This Florida doctor is cited in Link, *Paradox of Southern Progressivism*, 158. Hardy and Pynchon include a photograph of children with hookworm, illustrating poor-looking children with bare and dirty feet, in *Millstones and Milestones*, 21.

34. Graves, "Divine Guidance."

35. Graves, "Divine Guidance." For the Pentecostal Church of God's beliefs in the role of faith and sickness see Mickey Crews, *The Church of God: A Social History* (Knoxville: University of Tennessee Press, 1990), 80–83.

36. Graves, "Divine Guidance."

37. In 1940 Goggans became a member of the National Committee on Maternal and Child Health. She was appointed by Frances Perkins, the US secretary of labor, and went on to a distinguished career as a regional nursing consultant for the Children's Bureau and subsequently the Maternal Child Services of the US Department of Health Education and Welfare. "Information about Lalla Mary Goggans," 1972, Biographical Material folder, box 37, MSC 330, ACNM Records.

38. Jule Graves, note, first line "On Jack's Creek," October 1954, Midwifery file, Straight Collection.

39. Jule Graves, note, first line "After an inspection of the eyes of school children," n.d., Midwifery file, Straight Collection.

40. Kirkland, "Memory Jewels," 10. Prior to 1950 the general public referred to Florida Indians as Seminoles. There were, however, two distinct tribes speaking two distinct languages. The Seminole Tribe of Florida Indians was federally recognized in 1957 and the Miccosukee Tribe of Indians of Florida in 1961. Patsy West, *The Seminole and Miccosukee Tribes of Southern Florida* (Charleston, SC: Arcadia, 2001), 8; Mrs. Frank Stranahan, "Report of Seminole Indian Committee Conservation Department," *FFWC Yearbook, 1918–1919*, 115–116.

41. Julia A. Hanson, "Division of Seminole Indians," *FFWC Yearbook, 1926–1927*, 129–130. The Seminole Indian Association of Florida was incorporated in 1913.

42. For a brief note on Conrad's arrival see James W. Covington, *The Seminoles of Florida* (Gainesville: University Press of Florida, 1993), 232; Harry A. Kersey Jr., *The Florida Seminoles and the New Deal, 1933–1942* (Boca Raton: Florida Atlantic, 1989), 7.

43. Molly Ladd-Taylor, *Mother-Work: Women, Child Welfare, and the State, 1890–1930* (Urbana: University of Chicago, 1994), 181.

44. Patsy West, a historian of the Seminole and Miccosukee Indians, notes that the tradition of naming children after white friends was not uncommon among Seminoles within a limited set of white people they befriended. In Betty Mae Tiger and Patsy West, *A Seminole Legend: The Life of Betty Mae Tiger* (Gainesville: University Press of Florida, 2001), 39.

45. Harvey Burnett, in Kirkland, "Memory Jewels," 11. Harvey Burnett was the president of the Florida Public Health Association in 1964.

46. "The Seminole Indian Association of Florida, Incorporated 1913 Order Book," September 8, 1933, W. Stanley Hanson Collection, Seminole/Miccosukee Photographic Archives of Florida, courtesy of Patsy West.

47. Goggans, "Wonderful Years," 9. Goggans named nine of the counties: Bay, Washington, Jackson, Franklin, Gulf, Liberty, Calhoun, Gadsden, and Wakulla. The headquarters was in Marianna, Jackson County.

48. Although Goggans notes that Graves and Ely helped her the most, she also worked with Clio McLaughlin, Frances Holly, and Mary Dodd. Goggans, "Wonderful Years," 9.

49. Goggans, "Wonderful Years," 6–7.

50. Smith, *Sick and Tired*, 129; Ladd-Taylor, "'Grannies' and 'Spinsters,'" 264; Wertz and Wertz, *Lying In*, 214.

51. Mary Beth Chambers, interview by Debra Ann Susie, March 1984, in Susie, *In the Way of Our Grandmothers*, 149.

52. Mary Lee Jones, interview by Debra Ann Susie, April 28, 1984, in Susie *In the Way of Our Grandmothers*, 180.

53. Goggans, "Wonderful Years," 7.

54. Unidentified midwife, in Susie, *In the Way of Our Grandmothers*, 46.

55. S. Smith, *Sick and Tired*, 129–139; Ladd-Taylor, "My Work Came out of Agony"; Susie, *In the Way of Our Grandmothers*, 46.

56. Jones, interview by Susie, 172.

57. Goggans, "Wonderful Years," 6–7.

58. Goggans, "Wonderful Years," 7.

59. Barney, *Authorized to Heal*, 113.

60. Dr. Joseph De Lee had advocated for the use of forceps in the new field of obstetrics, but he retracted that recommendation in the mid-1920s and blamed himself and his colleagues for the spread of infections and a high maternal death rate. He noted that the childbirth conducted by physicians and obstetricians in hospitals was detrimental to mothers' health and therefore advocated home births. Judith Walzer Leavitt, *Brought to Bed: Child-Rearing in America, 1750–1950* (New York: Oxford University Press, 1986), 179–187.

61. Goggans, "Wonderful Years," 7.

62. Lucile Spire Blachly, "Prelude—Child Hygiene," *Florida Health Notes* 22, no. 4 (April 1930): 52. See also Lucille Spire Blachly, "Midwife Survey, 1931," *Florida Health Notes* 23, no. 2 (1931): 44.

63. Henry Hanson (1877–1954) began his career in Florida in 1909 as the director of the board's Division of Bacteriologic Laboratories. He served in the US Army Medical Corps during World War I in Panama. After the war he was employed by the Rockefeller Foundation to address public health issues in Peru. He was the state health officer in Florida from 1929 to 1935 and from 1942 to 1945. Henry Hanson, *The Pied Piper of Peru* (Jacksonville, FL: Convention, 1961). See also Hardy and Pynchon, "Henry Hanson," in *Millstones and Milestones*, 40–41.

64. Henry Hanson, "Report to Dr. H. Mason Smith, President of the State Board of Health, January 1, 1933," in *Decade in Public Health*, vii.

65. Blachly, "Midwife Survey, 1931," 44–45.

66. Blachly, "Midwife Survey, 1931," 44.

67. Blachly, "Midwife Survey, 1931," 44–45.

68. Henry Hanson and Lucile Spire Blachly, "Present Status of Midwifery In Florida," *Southern Medical Journal* 25, no. 12 (December 1932): 1252–1258.

69. For Blachly's announcement see "Midwife Survey, 1931," 44.

70. Goggans, "Wonderful Years," 5.

71. Hanson and Blachly, "Present Status of Midwifery in Florida."

72. Goggans, "Wonderful Years," 5.

73. Section 3, Act Relating to the Public Health and to the Control and Licensing of Midwifery for the Protection of Mothers at Childbirth, Laws of Florida, *General Acts and Resolutions adopted by the Legislature of Florida*, vol. 1, 1931, p. 471.

74. Goggans enlisted the help of a judge in West Palm Beach who was a friend of the family. She prepared a draft that was submitted to Hanson and the legal adviser to the State Board of Health. Within a year the bill became law. Goggans, "Wonderful Years," 9–10; Joyce Ely, untitled transcript of a talk possibly to the FFWC, ca. 1934, file folder 1, carton 1, series 904, Midwife Program Files, Florida State Archives.

75. Goggans, "Wonderful Years," 5.

76. Jones, interview by Susie, 177.

77. Graves, back of the photograph *African American Midwife Wearing a Protective Mask,* ca. 1940, black-and-white photoprint, 5 × 3 inches, State Archives of Florida, Florida Memory, https://www.floridamemory.com/items/show/44606.

78. Goggans, "Wonderful Years," 5.

79. The two nurses who remained with Ely when the State Board of Health suspended the nursing department were Mary G. Dodd, assigned to tuberculosis work, and Annie Gabriel, assigned to communicable diseases. "Report of the Division of Public Health Nursing, 1932," in *Decade in Public Health*, 64.

80. H. Hanson, "Report to Dr. H. Mason Smith," vii.

81. Joyce Ely, January–September; Lalla Mary Goggans, August–December; Jule O. Graves, September–December; Mary G. Dodd, January–December; Annie Gabriel, January–December, "Report of the Division of Public Health Nursing, 1932," in *Decade in Public Health*, 64.

82. Henry Hanson, "Report to Dr. N. A. Baltzell, President, State Board of Health," December 31, 1933, in *State Board of Health of Florida Thirty-Fourth Annual Report, 1933* (Jacksonville: State Board of Health, 1934), 4.

83. Ely left on September 15, 1932. "Report of the Division of Public Health Nursing, 1932," 64. Certificate awarded July 31, 1933, to Joyce Ely, Honor Roll, box 12, ACNM Records.

84. Goggans, "Wonderful Years," 10. No communication survived.

85. Goggans, "Wonderful Years" 10.

86. Goggans, "Wonderful Years," 10; Graves, "Midwife Program in Florida," *Public Health Nursing*, 527; Hardy and Pynchon, *Millstones and Milestones*, 135.

87. Goggans, "Wonderful Years," 11. County health departments in Florida grew in the 1930s. Taylor County in the Panhandle was the first to establish a county health unit, in 1930, followed by Leon in 1931 and Escambia in 1932. Wilson T. Sowder, "The Growth of Local Health Units in Florida," *Public Health Reports* 68, no. 11 (November 1953): 1083–1085; "Extent of Rural Health Services in the United States, December 31, 1932, to December 31, 1936," *Public Health Reports* 52, no. 47 (November 19, 1937): 1643.

88. In Lalla Mary Goggans, "Florida's First Institute for Midwives," paper presented to Florida State Nurses Association, St. Petersburg, Florida, 1933, General Contents folder, box 34, Lalla Mary Goggins [*sic*] Collection, ACNM Records.

89. Goggans, "Wonderful Years," 11. See also "Outline of Midwife Program," in "Division of Public Health Nursing," in *State Board of Health of Florida Thirty-Fourth Annual Report, 1933*, 51–52.

90. "Lalla Mary Goggins" [*sic*], Biographical Material folder, box 37, MSC 330, ACNM Records.

91. Goggans became the state nurse supervisor in Local Health Services before heading to Teachers College in 1938 for advanced courses in public health and midwifery. Goggans, "Wonderful Years," 13.

92. Graves, "Midwife Program in Florida," unpublished manuscript, 1–5.

93. "Report of the Division of Public Health Nursing," 1933, *State Board of Health of Florida Thirty-Fourth Annual Report*, 54.

94. The State Board of Health annual report for 1933 draws on figures relating to the 1930 survey. It states that of the 1,552 midwives in Florida, 50 percent had complied with the law and were licensed. There was no law at the time of the survey. The survey refers to the State Board of Health certificate of fitness. Of the 736 licensed and registered midwives, 11 percent were white and 89 percent black. Of the 789 who were not licensed, 20 percent were white and 80 percent black. "Report of the Division of Public Health Nursing," 1933, *State Board of Health of Florida Thirty-Fourth Annual Report*, 54.

95. Brown, "Experiment That Won Permanency."

96. Goggans, "Wonderful Years," 10.

97. Ruth E. Mettinger, in "Report of the Division of Public Health Nursing," *State Board of Health of Florida Thirty-Fifth Annual Report, 1934* (Jacksonville: State Board of Health, 1935), 45.

98. Goggans, "Wonderful Years," 11–12.

99. "Mrs. Ethel Jones Kirkland RN MPH CNM: Florida Public Health Association Meritorious Service Award," Honor Roll, box 11, 1971, ACNM Records.

100. Sowder to Straight, December 1, 1980. Sowder explained that a sawed-off shotgun in the era of Al Capone and gangsters was the equivalent of carrying a machine gun. In 1934 the National Firearm Act was signed into law to eliminate the weapons popular with gangsters such as machine guns and short-barrel shotguns like the one Graves possessed.

101. Kirkland, "Memory Jewels," 14

102. Jule O. Graves to Emil Davidson, vice president of Clay-Adams Company Inc., New York, June 15, 1951. Graves explains the origins of making the manikin, its purpose, and the possible advantages of its future manufacture and sale. Graves spent approximately $800 to secure the patent. File 9, carton 1, series 904, Midwife Program Files, Florida State Archives.

103. Graves, "Midwife Program in Florida," 6; Kirkland, "Memory Jewels," 14.

104. Kirkland, "Memory Jewels," 3, 4.

105. Jule O. Graves, "Midwife Program in Florida," unpublished manuscript, 3.

106. Lalla Mary Goggans, caption to a photograph of Jule Graves, Biographical Material folder, box 37, MSC 330, ACNM Records.

Chapter 5. Battling On without Fanfare for Better Health Conditions, 1934 to 1964

1. Ruth E. Mettinger, "Must 'Ration' Nurses, Too," *Florida Health Notes* 35, no. 4 (April 1943): 79.

2. "Nursing Service: Application for Enrollment," Mettinger, Ruth Esther, Historical Nurse files, box 62, ANRC Records.

3. Nannie J. Minor, Supt, Instructive Visiting Nurse Association, Richmond, Virginia, "Notation," June 4, 1918. Mettinger registered in Pennsylvania on March 28, 1916, and in Florida on June 8, 1916. Application to Red Cross Nursing Service, March 23, 1917, Mettinger, Ruth Esther, Mettinger, Historical Nurse Files.

4. H. Hanson, "State Health Officer's Report," in *Decade in Public Health*, 10.

5. American Public Health Association, "The Health Situation in Florida," report, January–June 1939, 7, Midwifery file, Straight Collection.

6. On the establishment and growth of the county health unit see Wilson T. Sowder, "The Growth of Local Health Units in Florida, *Public Health Reports* 68, no. 11 (November 1953): 1083–1088; Hardy and Pynchon, *Millstones and Milestones*, 65–74; David L. Crane, "Development of the Florida County Public Health System," *Journal of the Florida Medical Association* 73, no. 4 (1986): 286–288.

7. W. H. Y. Smith, "Birth and the Early Days of Florida's First County Health Unit," *Public Health Reports* 68, no. 11 (November 1953): 1088–1090.

8. In W. Smith, "Birth and the Early Days," 1088.

9. W. Smith, "Birth and the Early Days," 1089.

10. W. Smith, "Birth and the Early Days," 1089.

11. W. Smith, "Birth and the Early Days," 1090.

12. Hardy and Pynchon, *Millstones and Milestones*, 68.

13. Hardy and Pynchon, *Millstones and Milestones*, 68–69.

14. Martha Stetson, "From an Interview with Mrs. Martha Stetson (Holloway), R.N. (Retired), at Her Home in St. Petersburg, Florida, June 1973," interview by Frederick Eberson in his book *Early Medical History of Pinellas Peninsula: A Quadricentennial Epoch* (St. Petersburg, FL: Valkyrie, 1973), 73–76. Eberson uses the Stetson interview (but not exclusively) in his book chapter "Public Health in Pinellas County." In a news article Stetson refers to granulated eyelids, blepharitis, a bacterial infection likely caused by poor hygiene. Nancy Osgood, "For 34 Years, a Job Well Done," *St. Petersburg Times*, August 1, 1956.

15. Stetson, interview by Eberson, 75.

16. Link, *Paradox of Southern Progressivism*, 221; Lynne S. Wilcox, "Worms and Germs, Drink and Dementia: US Health, Society, and Policy in the Early 20th Century," *Preventing Chronic Disease: Public Health Research, Practice, and Policy* 5, no. 4 (October 2008): 3–4.

17. Stetson, interview by Eberson, 75.

18. Stetson, interview by Eberson, 76–77; Martha Stetson, "Guiding the Midwives," *Florida Health Notes* 7, no. 1 (January 1945): 13–15.

19. Henry Hanson, "State Health Officer's Report," in *State Board of Health of Florida Thirty-Fifth Annual Report, 1934* (Jacksonville: State Board of Health, 1935), 5.

20. H. Hanson, "Report to Dr. N. A. Baltzell," 5.

21. "Report of the Bureau of Child Hygiene and Public Health Nursing," 1930, in *Decade in Public Health*, 57.

22. Ruth E. Mettinger, "Effect of the ERA Nursing Services on Volunteer and Official Agencies," *American Journal of Public Health* 26, no. 7 (July 1936), 686.

23. Ruth E. Mettinger, "Public Health Nursing Standards," *Florida Health Notes* 26, no. 11 (November 1934): 165.

24. Ruth E. Mettinger, "CWA Nursing Program," *Florida Health Notes* 26, no. 5 (May 1934): 68–69.

25. Ruth E. Mettinger, "FERA Institute at Tampa," *Florida Health Notes* 16, no. 6 (June 1934): 84–85.

26. Mettinger, "FERA Institute at Tampa," 34–35.

27. Henry Hanson, "Administration," *Florida Health Notes* 26, no. 5 (May 1934): 68.

28. Mettinger, "Public Health Nursing Standards," 165.

29. Ruth E. Mettinger, "Public Health Councils," *Florida Health Notes* 29, no. 1 (January 1937): 5.

30. Mettinger, "Public Health Councils," 5.

31. Ruth E. Mettinger, "Report for Division of Public Health Nursing," in *State Board of Health of Florida Thirty-Sixth Annual Report, 1935* (Jacksonville: State Board of Health, 1936), 42.

32. Ruth E. Mettinger, "Progress of the E.R.A. Nursing Service," *Florida Health Notes* 27, no. 1 (January 1935): 42–43.

33. Mettinger, "Public Health Councils," 5. See also Ruth E. Mettinger, "Public Health Nursing," in *State Board of Health of Florida Fortieth Annual Report, 1939* (Jacksonville: State Board of Health, 1939), 40; Dolores M. Wennlund, *Annals of Public Health Nursing in Florida* (Tallahassee: State Public Health Office, 1992), 12.

34. Mettinger, "Public Health Nursing," 1939, 41.

35. American Public Health Association, "Health Situation in Florida," 38; F. V. Chappell, "Bureau of Maternal and Child Health," in *State Board of Health of Florida Thirty-Eighth Annual Report, 1937* (Jacksonville: State Board of Health, 1938), 132–133.

36. Clio McLaughlin, "Post-Sanatorium Care," *Florida Health Notes* 30, no. 12 (December 1938): 187; A. J. Logie, "The Status of Tuberculosis in Florida," *Florida Health Notes* 30, no. 12 (December 1938): 179; Ruth E. Mettinger, "Nursing Field Work in Tuberculosis," *Florida Health Notes* 29, no. 12 (December 1937): 190–191.

37. Logie, "Status of Tuberculosis in Florida," 178.

38. Logie, "Status of Tuberculosis in Florida," 179–181.

39. W. A. McPhaul, "County Tuberculosis Sanitariums," *Florida Health Notes* 30, no. 12 (December 1938): 177.

40. Lantana Hospital opened in 1950 with 500 beds, Tampa in 1951 with 550 beds, and Tallahassee in 1958 with 1,850 beds. Manni, "History of Tuberculosis in Florida," 308.

41. Manni, "History of Tuberculosis in Florida," 308.

42. American Public Health Association, "Health Situation in Florida," 46.

43. American Public Health Association, "Health Situation in Florida," 46.

44. In "Public Health Nursing: Ruth E. Mettinger R.N. Director of Nursing," *Florida Health Notes* 31, no. 1–2 (January 1939): 5.

45. Higgs, interview, October 22, 1997; "Homegoing Services for Mother Grace M. Higgs," program, Mt. Zion Missionary Baptist Church, Miami, June 20, 1998. Author's Public Health Nursing file.

46. In Thomas, *Deluxe Jim Crow*, 62–68. See also Parran, "Public Health Marches On," 86–90.

47. In Thomas, *Deluxe Jim Crow*, 63.

48. Ruth Stuart Allen, "A Visit to the Rapid Treatment Center," *Florida Health Notes* 40, no. 2 (February 1948): 35. Until penicillin was mass-produced in the 1940s, syphilis was treated with Salvarsan, an arsenic-based drug developed by Paul Ehrlich in 1908.

49. Born in Jacksonville, Okel V. Welsh was one of the nurses who enrolled in the Cadet Nurse Corps and received her nursing education at Grady Hospital Training School in Atlanta. After the war she returned to Florida and in 1947 accepted employment at the Rapid Treatment Center. Okel V. Welsh, interview by the author, June 6, 1997, Miami.

50. Ruth E. Mettinger, "The Public Health Nurse in the Control of Syphilis," *Florida Health Notes* 30, no. 2 (February 1938): 23.

51. Mettinger, "Public Health Nurse in the Control of Syphilis," 23.

52. Mettinger, "Public Health Nurse in the Control of Syphilis," 24.

53. Mettinger, "Public Health Nurse in the Control of Syphilis," 24.

54. F. V. Chappell, "Prevent Syphilitic Babies," *Florida Health Notes* 30, no. 2 (February 1938): 25.

55. Mettinger, "Public Health Nurse in the Control of Syphilis," 23. See also Thomas, *Deluxe Jim Crow*, 62–68.

56. Mettinger, "Public Health Nurse in the Control of Syphilis," 23.

57. "Ignorance and Quacks Take Heavy Toll among Negroes; Units Attacking Problem," *Florida Health Notes* 32, no. 4 (April 1940): 58.

58. "Ignorance and Quacks Take Heavy Toll among Negroes," 58.

59. Allen, "Visit to the Rapid Treatment Center," 31.

60. "Ignorance and Quacks Take Heavy Toll among Negroes," 58.

61. Wilson T. Sowder to William M. Straight, December 1, 1980, Midwifery file, Straight Collection.

62. Sowder to Straight, December 1, 1980.

63. "Mrs. Ethel Jones Kirkland RN MPH CNM: Florida Public Health Association Meritorious Service Award," Honor Roll, box 11, 1971, ACNM Records.

64. Sowder to Straight, December 1, 1980.

65. Sowder to Straight, December 1, 1980.

66. Ruth E. Mettinger, "Bureau of Public Health Nursing," in *State Board of Health of Florida Thirty-Seventh Annual Report, 1936* (Jacksonville: State Board of Health, 1937), 48.

67. In "Mrs. Ethel Jones Kirkland RN MPH CNM." See also Goggans, "Wonderful Years," 11–12.

68. Mettinger, "Bureau of Public Health Nursing," 1936, 49.

69. Mettinger, "Public Health Nursing," 1939, 44.

70. Mettinger, "Public Health Nursing," 1939, 43.

71. Ruth E. Mettinger, "Public Health Nursing," in *State Board of Health of Florida Forty-Third Annual Report, 1942* (Jacksonville: State Board of Health, 1943), 159.

72. Ruth E. Mettinger, "Public Health Nursing," in *State Board of Health of Florida Forty-Second Annual Report, 1941* (Jacksonville: State Board of Health, 1942), 159.

73. Ruth E. Mettinger, "Bureau of Public Health Nursing," in *State Board of Health of Florida Forty-Fourth Annual Report, 1943* (Jacksonville: State Board of Health, 1944), 213.

74. Ruth E. Mettinger, "Bureau of Public Health Nursing," in *State Board of Health of Florida Forty-Sixth Annual Report, 1945* (Jacksonville: State Board of Health, 1946), 87.

75. Ruth E. Mettinger, "Bureau of Public Health Nursing," in *State Board of Health of Florida Forty-Ninth Annual Report, 1948* (Jacksonville: State Board of Health, 1949), 94.

76. Ruth E. Mettinger, "Division of Public Health Nursing," in *State Board of Health of Florida Fifty-Third Annual Report, 1952* (Jacksonville: State Board of Health, 1953), 65.

77. Mettinger, "Division of Public Health Nursing," 1952, 65.

78. Ruth E. Mettinger, "Division of Public Health Nursing," in *State Board of Health of Florida Sixty-First Annual Report, 1960* (Jacksonville: State Board of Health, 1961), 39.

79. L. L. Parks, "Bureau of Maternal and Child Health," in *State Board of Health of Florida Sixty-First Annual Report, 1960*, 85–88. The statistical chart in Parks's report is "Resident Maternal Death Rate (per 10,000 Live Births) by Race, Florida, 1935–1960," 86.

80. Ruth E. Mettinger, "Division of Public Health Nursing," in *State Board of Health of Florida, Sixty-Third Annual Report, 1962* (Jacksonville: State Board of Health, 1963), 38.

81. Susie, *In The Way of Our Grandmothers*, 49.

82. In Charlotte Downey-Anderson, "The 'Coggins Affair': Desegregation and Southern Mores in Madison County, Florida," *Florida Historical Quarterly* 59, no. 4 (April 1981): 466.

83. Sowder to Straight, December 1, 1980.

84. The Associated Press stories ran under those headlines in the *Seattle Daily News*, September 19 and 28, 1956.

85. "Health Officer Firing Criticized by Governor," *Aberdeen* (SD) *Daily News*, September 1956, 2.

86. "Cowards! Lady Gets Last Word on Firing," *Dallas Morning News*, October 4, 1956, 1.

87. Downey-Anderson, "The 'Coggins Affair,'" 464-472.

88. Sowder to Straight, December 1, 1980.

89. Sowder to Straight, December 1, 1980.

90. Betty Hilliard, oral history interview by Ann Smith, February 2, 2001, 57, Sam Proctor Oral History Program Collection, P. K. Yonge Library of Florida History, University of Florida, Gainesville.

91. Hilliard, interview by Smith.

92. Thelma Anderson Gibson, interview by the author, March 3, 1995, Miami; Idella Hogan, interview by the author, March 5, 1995, Miami.

93. "Newsreel: Florida," *National News Bulletin* 12, no. 2 (August 1939), NACGN records.

94. In Gillies, "[Long] History of the Florida Nurses Association," 117.

95. In Gillies, "[Long] History of the Florida Nurses Association," 117.

96. The associations in Delaware, Florida, and Maryland opened to racial integration in 1943. For a concise summary see Mabel K. Staupers, "Story of the National Association of Colored Graduate Nurses," *American Journal of Nursing* 51, no. 4, (April 1951): 223.

97. Carnegie, *Path We Tread*, 81.

98. Gillies, "[Long] History of the Florida Nurses Association," 137.

99. Mary Elizabeth Carnegie, "The Impact of Integration on the Nursing profession: An Historical Sketch," *Negro History Bulletin* 28, no. 7 (April 1965): 154–155.

100. Gillies, "[Long] History of the Florida Nurses Association," 137.

101. Carnegie, *Path We Tread*, 81.

102. The American Nurses Association's platform is cited in M. Patricia Donahue, *Nursing, the Finest Art* (St. Louis, MO: Mosby, 1985), 369. On the dissolution of the National Associa-

tion of Colored Graduate Nurses See Carnegie, *Path We Tread*, 107–109; Hine, *Black Women in White*, 185–186.

103. In Thelma Anderson Gibson, Helen McGuire, and Howard Carter, *Forebearance: Thelma Vernall Anderson Gibson; The life Story of a Cocoanut Grove Native* (Homestead, FL: Helena Enterprises, 2000), 138.

104. In Gibson, McGuire, and Carter, *Forebearance*, 137–138.

105. In Gibson, McGuire, and Carter, *Forebearance*, 142.

106. Parran, "Public Health Marches On," 90.

Conclusion: Tracing Footprints from the Past

1. In 1969 the State Board of Health was abolished, and public health functioned as an administrative division under the Department of Health and Rehabilitative Services (HRS). In 1975 the HRS Reorganization Act passed to further decentralize and unify the provision of health, rehabilitative, and social services. Bigler, "Public Health in Florida," 23.

2. "Racial Disparities in Tuberculosis, 1991–2002," *CDC Morbidity and Mortality Weekly Report* 53, no. 25 (July 2, 2004): 556–559, https://www.cdc.gov/mmwr/preview/mmwrhtml/mm5325a3.htm; Cecilia Rivera Casale, "Disparities in Healthcare Quality among Racial and Ethnic Minority Groups," selected findings from *2010 National Healthcare Quality and Disparities Reports*, Agency of Healthcare Research and Quality, US Department of Health and Human Services.

3. McBride, *From TB to AIDS*, 170. McBride's study offers parallels to the impact of Florida's neglect of black citizens' health care as well as a failure of American medicine. Darlene Clark Hine reiterates as much in "Taking Care of Bodies, Babies, and Business: Black Women Health Professionals in South Carolina, 1895–1954," in *Writing Women's History: A Tribute to Anne Firor Scott*, ed. Elizabeth Anne Payne (Jackson: University Press of Mississippi, 2011), 123.

4. McBride, *From TB to AIDS*, 171.

5. Carnegie, *Path We Tread*, 128.

6. Carnegie, *Path We Tread*, 127.

7. Brown, speech to International Council of Nurses convention in Germany, 1911; Beckett, "Of Interest to Nurses."

8. Carnegie, *Path We Tread*, 127–128. See also "History," National Black Nurses Association, n.d., https://www.nbna.org/history.

9. Community-based programs included preventive health screenings and health education. "Who We Are," National Black Nurses Association, October 24, 2013, https://www.nbna.org/who.

10. Dolores M. Wennlund, interview by the author, February 4, 2010, Lutz, FL; Kim Curry, "Dolores Wennlund, Florida Public Health Nursing Leader: A Career Journey," Florida Public Health Association, n.d., http://www.fpha.org/Resources/Documents/FAPHN.DoloresWennlund.pdf, accessed May 26, 2018.

11. Wennlund, *Annals of Public Health Nursing in Florida*, 32.

12. Buhler-Wilkinson, "False Dawn," 100–101. See also Karen Buhler-Wilkinson, "Public Health Then and Now, Bringing Care to People: Lillian Wald's Legacy to Public Health Nursing," *American Journal of Public Health* 83, no. 12 (December 1993): 1778–1786.

13. Wennlund, interview by the author.

14. Wennlund, *Annals of Public Health Nursing in Florida*, 90.

15. Laurie Jean Reid to Grace Abbott, March 7, 1923, file 4-10-4-0, box 190, RG 102, CB Central File, 1921–24.

16. "Mrs. Ethel Jones Kirkland RN, MPH, CNM," ACNM Records.

17. Jane Wilcox, "Public Health Nursing Section," in *Division of Health Annual Report for Florida, 1972* (Tallahassee: HRS State Health Office, 1973): 41–42.

18. Paul Starr, *The Social Transformation of American Medicine* (New York: Basic Books, 1982), 265, 283; Thomas, *Deluxe Jim Crow*, 100.

19. Starr, *Social Transformation of American Medicine*, 350, 389.

20. Johnnie Seeley, interview by Debra Ann Susie, April 1982, in Susie, *In the Way of Our Grandmothers*, 128.

21. Wilcox, "Public Health Nursing Section," 41–42.

22. Wennlund, *Annals of Public Health Nursing in Florida*, 37, 58, 73–74, 88.

23. Schools to train traditional midwives grew in Florida. In 1992 and again in 1995 the Midwifery Practice Act was updated to ensure qualifications and authorize licensing. Some states allow certified nurse midwives to work independently; Florida does not.

24. Wennlund, *Annals of Public Health Nursing in Florida*, 74.

25. Crista Craven and Mara Glotzel, "Downplaying Difference: Historical Accounts of African American Midwives and Contemporary Struggles for Midwifery," *Feminist Studies* 36, no. 2 (Summer 2010): 330–358.

26. Augusta Wilson, interview by Debra Ann Susie, August 6, 1981, in Susie, *In the Way of Our Grandmothers*, 77. See also Annie Mae Taylor, interview by Peggy A. Bulger, June 6, 1979, North Florida Folklife Project, audio transcript S1576,T79-5, Florida Memory, https://floridamemory.com.

27. Michael C. Lu, Milton Kotelchuck, Vijaya, Loretta Jones, Kynna Wright, and Neal Halfon, "Closing the Black-White Gap in Birth Outcomes: A Life Course Approach," *Ethnicity and Disease* 20, no. 102 (Winter 2010): 62–76; Holly Mead, Lara Cartwright-Smith, Karen Jones, Christal Ramos, Kristy Woods, and Bruce Siegel, "Disparities in Health Status and Mortality," in *Racial and Ethnic Disparities in U.S. Healthcare: A Chartbook*, 19–30 (n.p.: Commonwealth Fund, March 2008), https://www.commonwealthfund.org/publications/publication/2008/mar/racial-and-ethnic-disparities-us-health-care-chartbook.

28. See, for example, Michelle Norris, host, "Why Black Women, Infants Lag in Birth Outcomes," *All Things Considered*, National Public Radio, July 8, 2011; Shun Zhang, Kathryn Cardarelli, Ruth Shim, Jiali Ye, Karla L. Booker, and George Rust, "Racial Disparities in Economic and Clinical Outcomes of Pregnancy among Medicaid Recipients," *Journal of Maternal Child Health* 17, no. 8 (October 2013): 1518–1525.

29. Tyan Parker Dominguez, Christine Dunkel-Schetter, Laura M. Glynn, Calvin Hobel, and Curt Sandman, "Racial Differences in Birth Outcomes: The Role of General Pregnancy and Racism Stress," *Health Psychology* 27, no. 2 (March 2008): 194–203; Zoe Carpenter, "What's Killing American Black Infants? Racism Is Fueling a National Crisis," *The Nation*, February 15, 2017.

30. Wilson, interview by Susie, 77–78.

31. Wennlund, *Annals of Public Health Nursing in Florida*, 90 (quote); Wennlund, interview by the author.

32. Nancy L. Fahrenwald, Janette Y. Taylor, Shawn M. Kneipp, and Mary K. Canales, "Academic Freedom and Academic Duty to Teach Social Justice: A Perspective and Pedagogy for Public Health Nursing Faculty," *Public Health Nursing* 24, no. 2 (March–April, 2007): 190–197; Nancy Krieger and Anne-Emanuelle Birn, "A Vision of Social Justice as the Foundation of Public Health: Commemorating 150 Years of the Spirit of 1848," *American Journal of Public Health* 88, no. 11 (November 1998): 1603–1606.

Index

Page numbers in *italics* refer to illustrations.

With roots as an English nurse, Christine Ardalan has dedicated her academic career in the United States to researching, writing, and preserving nursing history. She is currently adjunct lecturer in American history at Florida International University.

CPSIA information can be obtained
at www.ICGtesting.com
Printed in the USA
BVHW030034290422
635320BV00001B/75

9 780813 068589